Dagmar-Pauline Heinke

Relieving Pain with
Acupressure

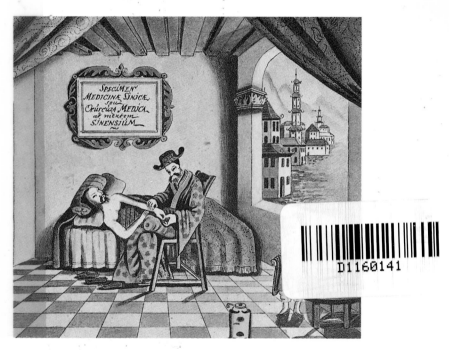

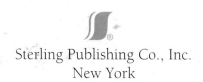

Sterling Publishing Co., Inc.
New York

Library of Congress
Cataloging-in-Publication Data

Heinke, Dagmar-Pauline.
  [Schmerzen Lindern mit
Akupressur. English]
Relieving pain with acupres-
sure / Dagmar-Pauline Heinke.
  p.   cm.
Includes index.
ISBN 0-8069-4213-4
1. Acupressure—Popular
works.
I. Title.
RM723.A27H4513 1998
615.8'22—dc21
98-40060
CIP

10 9 8 7 6 5 4 3 2 1

Published 1998 by Sterling
  Publishing Company, Inc.
  387 Park Avenue South,
  New York, N.Y. 10016
Originally published and © 1995 in
  Germany by Sudwest Verlag
  under the title *Schmerzen lindern
  mit Akupressur*
English translation © 1998 by
  Sterling Publishing Co., Inc.
Distributed in Canada by Sterling
  Publishing
  % Canadian Manda Group,
  One Atlantic Avenue, Suite 105
  Toronto, Ontario, Canada M6K 3E7
Distributed in Great Britain and
  Europe by Cassell PLC
  Wellington House, 125 Strand,
  London WC2R 0BB, England
Distributed in Australia by
  Capricorn Link (Australia) Pty Ltd.
  P.O. Box 6651, Baulkham Hills,
  Business Centre, NSW 2153,
  Australia
*Manufactured in the United States of
  America*
Sterling ISBN 0-8069-4213-4

Contents

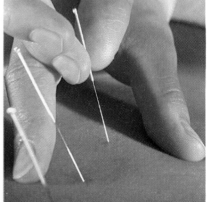

*Self-treatment with
acupressure*

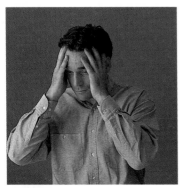

Do you often feel ill for no apparent reason?

For most of us, illness is a very unpleasant experience. Although we combat our aches and pains with potent medications, the cause of the problem frequently remains untreated.

The Philosophy of the Chinese Art of Healing

A Disruption of Harmony

In the West, whenever we feel ill or experience aches and pains, we want to fix the problem as fast as possible. That's why we are so quick to reach for pills, hoping that they will help us feel better immediately and make our pains disappear. We wait for these soothing results without giving any thought to the cause of the problem, how we may have contributed to it, or the interaction of mind and body.

Chinese medicine, on the other hand, does not merely treat symptoms, but is concerned with the source of the illness as well. The Chinese have a saying: "Every cause has its effect, and every effect its cause." This philosophy urges them to look for the root of the problem.

Different Cultures—Similar Principles

Hippocrates, the physician known as the father of medicine, spread similar ideas to those of the Chinese in ancient Greece, a culture very different from that of China. He assumed that the source of every illness was a disruption of harmony, and he was quite successful in

Harmonic Energy

Every one of our cells has its own special mode of expression, or its own "vibration spectrum."

Differing vibrations that meet and overlap can be weakened or strengthened. Intensified positive and har-monic energy vibrations nullify certain vibrations that can cause illness.

So, it follows that when we lose our inner harmony, we run a greater risk of becoming ill.

treating patients by restoring their balance. Interestingly, this is the very principle that forms the basis of Chinese medicine.

Health and Illness

When is a person healthy? According to the World Health Organization (WHO), a healthy person is completely well physically, mentally, psychologically, and socially. Thus, when all of our body parts are functioning properly, laboratory findings are normal, and we don't feel any pain or discomfort, and if we are fortunate enough to have an inner power and vitality and our life is harmonious on the outside as well, then we can truly say that we are healthy.

But how many people deceive themselves day after day, avoiding a confrontation with their emotional conflicts? How many keep up outward appearances, only to try to hide a life based on nothing more than an illusion? How many pretend that they are happy in their relations with others, but in reality are unhappy and burdened with anxiety?

Health is a holistic concept. This means that health is more than the flawless functioning of the body's organs and normal laboratory reports.

Enduring stress is part of the daily routine of many jobs. We tend to ignore the fact that stress can make us sick, even though we may not end up with a heart attack.

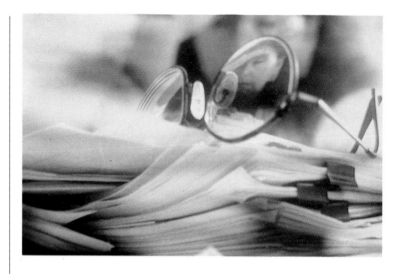

Complete health is inseparable from values like harmony, love, and contentment.

Health Means Wholeness

Are successful corporate managers who put on airs of competence and strength truly healthy? Think of the important decisions they have to make under enormous stress. And what happens as they slowly become estranged from their family?

A definition of health must take into account the whole body, the mind, and the soul. Among other things, a healthy person shows love, devotion, honesty, compassion, dependability, humility, modesty, contentment, and fairness. Although these virtues may seem old-fashioned, integrating them into our life helps keep us healthy and happy. They charge our aura with a positive energy that is reflected onto everyone around us. This harmony activates the self-healing powers of our body and makes us more resistant to illness.

Self-Healing Powers

☛ What is meant by this is that we activate the "physician within us."

☛ We can mobilize the healing powers within our body by using natural forms of therapy as well as positive thinking.

☛ We can return the body to balance and thus regain harmony.

A Lack of Balance

Examples of a lack of balance or harmony aren't hard to find. Think about what happens when a personal relationship ends: hate, mistrust, and rejection often replace love, trust, and devotion. These negative feelings carry a great deal of negative energy, which can affect the body and mind, opening the door to illness.

A Chance to Make Changes

Illness is caused by a disruption of harmony in your body, mind, and soul. Thus, we can define illness as an imbalance between the needs of your soul and your myriad reactions.

Although this loss of balance provokes illness, it also gives you the opportunity to make badly needed changes in your life . The corporate manager who suffers a heart attack now has a chance to reflect on his or her life and perhaps reorder priorities. If you are unhappy in a personal relationship and keeping your emotions bottled up inside, you might have an accident and break a leg, which will give you time to think about how you are handling your situation.

The cause of many illnesses can be traced back to the mind. Today, this concept is generally accepted. If we view illness as a chance to make needed changes, we have an opportunity to create a positive outcome.

A positive outlook not only helps us overcome illnesses, but also allows us to recognize the opportunities that illnesses offer to make changes in our lives.

Changing Ourselves

When we try to analyze ourselves in relation to the world around us, we should look at both our strengths and our weaknesses. Our aim must be to change ourselves and not others.

This will lead to a greater knowledge of ourselves and a more tolerant attitude toward others. It also will open the way to taking more responsibility and having a greater ability to help others.

Facing Up to Reality

Every illness is the body's attempt to rid itself of excessive negative energy and destructive potential. The main problem is always a psychological one. We have to find out what or whom is obstructing us, which is usually very difficult because we tend to suppress everything we don't like. We have a hard time facing ourselves and accepting reality.

Your Health Is Your Own Decision!

Sooner or later, we are bound to become ill because of the negative influences in life. We all experience disappointments and conflicts as well as victories and successes. However, what we experience depends to a large extent on how we interpret it. We can say that a glass is half full, or we can say that it is half empty. The main key to the doors of health in our body and our mind is found in having a positive attitude toward life, one that focuses on what is important and good for us.

The Psychological Causes of Illness

Illness can be a turning point. We need to recognize where we may have gone wrong and correct the problems in our lifestyle. Frustrations and negative thoughts poison our feelings. Sooner or later, this leads to an illness, which is a reflection of its underlying psychological causes.

Man—a Reflection of the Cosmos

Thousands of years ago, the Chinese learned about life by closely observing nature and its laws. They studied the seasons, climates, colors, and time. Chinese medicine is based on a holistic approach whereby the microcosm, man, is viewed as a reflection of the macrocosm and, therefore, is subject to the same laws that govern it.

It's important to treat the illness or the affected organ, but we also must get to the root of the illness and find the cause of the disharmony. Only by so doing can the patient be cured successfully. The chart on pages 10 and 11 is a brief overview of the most common disorders and their psychological causes.

Man does not exist in isolation. We are a part of, and reflect, the intricate pattern of the cosmos.

Illness as Opportunity

Illness always gives us an opportunity to recognize the truth, to make corrections in our lifestyle, and to change other bad habits.

Signals of Common Disorders

DISORDER	PSYCHOLOGICAL BASIS
Acne	Lack of self-esteem
Allergies	Defensiveness
Anorexia nervosa	Self-hate; sexual problems
Anxiety	Lack of confidence in one's own strength
Apathy	Resistance to emotions
Appetite problems	Fear of life
Asthma	Inability to act naturally; repression
Backache	Lack of love; lack of support; financial problems
Bed-wetting	Fear of parents or guardians; lack of love and affection
Bladder problems	Fear of letting go
Blood pressure, high	Mind working at full speed; many unsolved problems
Blood pressure, low	Inability to withstand stress; low self-esteem
Bone disorders	Pressure; strain; problems with authority
Bronchitis	Problems with family relationships; aggression
Colds	Retreat; pause; be fed up
Constipation	Clinging to the past; stinginess
Disk problems (backache)	Feeling abandoned
Ear problems	Unwillingness to listen
Eczema	Psychogenic resistance; suppressed conflicts
Genital problems	Self-doubt; guilt complex; suppressed sexuality
Hair loss	Stress; strain; worry
Hay fever	Pent-up feelings; anxiety
Headache	Anxiety; self-punishment

Signals of Common Disorders

DISORDER	PSYCHOLOGICAL BASIS
Heart complaints	Bleakness; emotional problems
Inflammation	Resistance to something; pent-up conflicts
Insomnia	Feelings of guilt; anxiety
Intestinal disorders	Trying to overcome problems in the subconscious
Kidney disorders	Disappointment; conflicts in relationships
Larynx, inflammation of	Speechless from rage
Leg problems	Fear of the future
Liver disorders	Resistance to new things; rage and negative feelings
Lung problems	Grief; depression
Menopause problems	Fear of not being attractive; fear of loneliness
Menstrual problems	Anxiety; rejection
Migraine	Suppressed anger
Neuritis	Pain as a punishment
Overweight	Defense against anxiety; self-rejection
Pancreas	Bitterness; disappointment
Premenstrual syndrome	Discontentment; unhappiness; mentally overtaxed
Rheumatism	Bitterness; lack of love
Sciatic pain	Fear of the future; money problems
Skin disorders	Emotional cry for help
Stomach disorders	Problems in accepting the truth; anxiety
Teeth (toothache)	Lack of ability to make decisions; aggression
Throat problems	Lack of ability to confront conflicts
Tonsillitis	Suppression; stifled creativity

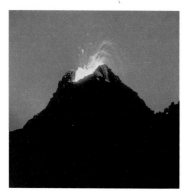

The power of the elements

Holism and Chinese Medicine

The Five Basic Elements

It is important to understand that the body is not just a machine operating on its own. It is constantly interacting with the mind and the soul. This is one of the underlying principles of Chinese medicine. Holism also is expressed in the Chinese concept of elemental principles, which forms the basis for the entire Chinese philosophy of life.

Learning about the five basic elements will help you better understand the principles of acupressure. Furthermore, they are closely related to the meridians, which are the points where you will start your self-treatment.

People in certain cultures relate to the basic elements in order to establish their position in the cosmos.

Religious Symbols

The five elements (earth, water, fire, metal, and wood) represent the bioenergetic principle. Many religions and cultures (such as those of Native Americans and the people of Tibet, Africa, India, and the Orient) look upon them as the prime components of creation.

The five elements are often an integral part of religious services and ceremonies. For example, in the Roman Catholic mass, candles represent the element of fire, incense symbolizes the element of metal, holy water stands for the element of water, and the consecrated wafers of the Host represent the element of earth.

Balance of the Elements

When people plan to build a house or furnish an apartment in China, the custom is to consult a special advisor in order to adhere strictly to the balance of the five elements. This way, the rooms will radiate harmony, having a positive effect on the inhabitants. Should one of the elements be lacking, they must add to it so that all of the elements are represented equally, thus avoiding disharmony.

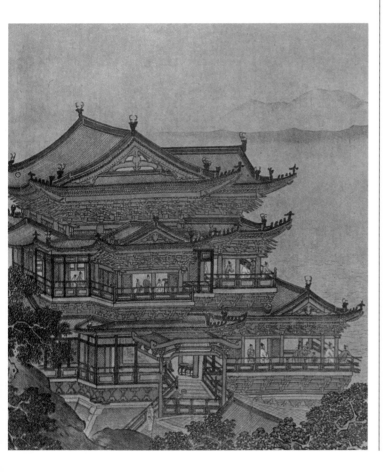

A house from the Sung Dynasty (A.D. 960 – 1279) in China, showing the high standards of Oriental architecture. When building such houses, the architect and the owner not only gave thought to appearance and usefulness, but they also took into consideration the harmonious balance of the five elements.

Harmonious Interaction

The principle of the five elements of wood, metal, fire, water, and earth is at the core of every Chinese science. No element is viewed in isolation, and in their interaction, each element can create another one:

☞ Wood burns and creates fire.

☞ Fire leaves ashes (earth).

☞ Earth is the source of metal.

☞ Metal can be turned into a liquid (water).

☞ Wood needs water to grow.

In this process, the preceding element always interacts in a positive way with the one that follows. Thus, we must adhere to the proper order during acupressure treatment in order to maintain harmony. Each of the five elements has an affinity for certain organs of the body, as well as for certain seasons, flavors, emotions, and the five senses. The

Every vital form is in continual states of growth and decay. Thus, any one element can evolve from another, and each one is linked to the others.

The Five Elements and Their Corresponding Organs

☞ Wood symbolizes life, femininity, and organic material; it is related to the liver and the gallbladder.

☞ Metal symbolizes masculinity, assertiveness, and material things; it is related to the lungs and the sense of touch.

☞ Fire symbolizes intelligence, energy, and warmth; it is related to the heart, the circulatory system, and the small intestines.

☞ Water symbolizes communication; it is related to the bladder, the kidneys, and the feet.

☞ Earth symbolizes form, strength, stability, and ruggedness; it is related to the stomach, the spleen, and the pancreas.

elements must remain in balance in order to guarantee a constant flow of vital energy and, therefore, maintain good health.

The Organs in Balance

The organs interact with each other in the same way as the five elements that they relate to do. Just as each element evolves from another, each organ has an organ that acts as a kind of "parent" to it. Whenever the "child" organ is ill, the "parent" organ needs treatment to support it. This is why, in addition to treating stomach pains through the stomach meridian, we also treat them through the spleen, pancreas, and circulation meridians.

The Polar Forces of Yin and Yang

Yin and yang symbolize the two polar body energies that complement each other and are in constant interaction. We are healthy if the yin and yang organs are in harmonious balance. A disrupted balance causes illness.

Yin and Yang—a Cosmic Principle of Life

According to the sixth-century B.C. Chinese philosopher Lao-tzu, the Tao is the unknowable source of all existence and the guiding principle of all reality. It is presented as a circle, symbolizing the limitlessness of existence, in which there is no beginning and no end.

Yin and yang, the masculine and feminine principles, fill this circle. They are represented by darkness and light, and interact in harmony with each other. The result is a harmonious and complete whole. In the dark part of the yin,

According to Chinese medicine, our organs interact in the same way as the five elements of nature do. For this reason, organs not directly affected by an illness also must be treated.

there is a little of the light part of the yang, and vice versa. This symbolizes that the two principles can never exist in isolation, but are always connected to their opposite pole.

One cannot exist without the other. There is some light in every darkness, and every end contains a new beginning. This means that illness and health are not isolated or opposite phenomena. They, too, represent the interaction between yin and yang.

The yin-yang symbol is the most well-known expression of wholeness in the Far East. Black and white, male and female, summer and winter, and good and bad all exist in mutual dependence, permeating and complementing each other.

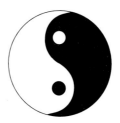

Vital Energy Through Yin and Yang

Chi to refers to the vital energy, or the energy of life, that flows through a special system of channels in our body. Chi flows unhindered when our body is healthy. But when Chi is blocked by disruptions, we don't feel well or we become ill.

The vital energy of Chi is composed of the polar forces of yin and yang. Think of yin and yang as being the opposite sides of a scale. Ideally, the sides should be in balance. When this is the case, the body is in harmony and is healthy.

When the equilibrium is disturbed, meaning that either yin or yang is stronger, we are in a state of disharmony, and we will become ill. The polar forces of yin and yang can be compared to:
☛ Summer and winter
☛ Male and female
☛ Life and death

The Yin and Yang Meridians

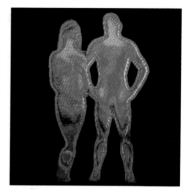

Energy flows through our body.

Chi, the vital energy of the body, flows through certain channels or pathways, called meridians. You can think of meridians as being somewhat like nerves. The body has 12 meridians, and they are always paired. Thus, there is a version of each meridian in the left half of the body as well as in the right half.

The meridians are divided into yin meridians and yang meridians. Understanding this division helps us comprehend our illnesses and treat them.

The Meridians			
Bladder	Yang	Liver	Yin
Circulation-sexuality	Yin	Lungs	Yin
Gallbladder	Yang	Small intestine	Yang
Heart	Yin	Spleen-pancreas	Yin
Kidney	Yin	Stomach	Yang
Large intestine	Yang	Triple warmer	Yang

The meridians are a complicated network of energy pathways running through our body. Chi, the energy of life, circulates within these pathways.

In addition, two special unpaired meridians, called vessels, run down the middle of the body: the conception vessel (yin) and the governing vessel (yang). The other special vessels need not concern us here. The aim of every treatment in Chinese medicine is to balance and harmonize the energy of the meridians.

All body organs have phases of activity and rest. The healing practices of the Far East make use of these alternating phases.

Conception Vessel—Jennmo (Receiver Vessel)

This special meridian starts at a point between the genitals and the anus, runs up past the abdomen, and ends at the chin. It is the communication vessel of the yin organs.

Governing Vessel—Toumo (Vessel of the Ruler)

Another special meridian, it starts in the gums and runs down the spine to the tip of the coccyx. It is connected to the yang organs. We treat all chronic, involuntary, and hormone-related illnesses through the governing vessel.

The energy of the conception vessel and the governing vessel is combined and forms a balance between yin and yang.

The Organic Clock

We know that the body changes in temperature. The changes are normal fluctuations that depend on the time of day. The fluctuations express oscillations of energy. Every meridian has phases of activity and rest, too. You can optimize the success of acupressure if you take the relevant times into account during treatment.

For example, the stomach zone's most active phase occurs between 8 and 10 o'clock in the morning. If you suffer from a nervous stomach condition, your stomach will be calmest during that time. If you want to stimulate this organ (perhaps because you suffer from a lack of appetite), you should treat the problem after 10 o'clock in the morning in order to lengthen the active phase. You will find the optimal times for treatment listed for each complaint.

TIP

This book indicates the best times for specific relaxing or stimulating therapy for every common complaint.

Acupressure and Acupuncture

The Oldest Healing Methods

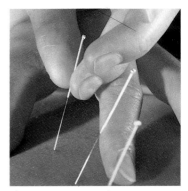

Acupuncture is painless, even though it uses needles.

Acupressure and acupuncture are healing methods that influence the flow of energy in the body by working on different meridians. With acupressure, you accomplish this with pressure from the fingers; with acupuncture, you use needles.

The Chinese have used acupressure and acupuncture for more than 6,000 years. Archaeological finds have confirmed its early practice. No other method of healing has such a long history with so many successes.

For years, people in the West were skeptical about this method of healing. Even today, many patients feel insecure the first time they are treated. They want to know whether or not acupuncture really works, or if it has just a placebo effect (if it only works if you believe it will work).

Acupressure and acupuncture act on certain points of the meridians. Thus, both methods of treatment influence the Chi, the flow of vital energy.

Even as Anesthesia

In Asia, the normal practice is to use acupuncture as an anesthetic during surgery. The great popularity that acupressure and acupuncture enjoy there is largely due to the understanding Asians have of themselves and of nature.

Acupuncture is nothing more than a development of acupressure. The needles enable us to work more precisely, and they go deeper under the skin.

Legend has it that Asians treated various forms of pain by rubbing the appropriate spots with their fingertips. This was the beginning of acupressure.

Subconsciously, we do the same thing, without even knowing anything about the techniques of acupressure. Think about what you do when you have a bad headache. Very often you will find yourself pressing your fingers on the painful spot on your temple or above your eyebrow. If you think about it, you will find many other examples of this kind of self-treatment.

From Acupressure to Acupuncture

Over the course of time, acupressure developed further. Documents dating back 2,000 years indicate that people were cured with the aid of bamboo sticks or rods made of bone. We don't know exactly when the change from using fingertips to using more effective and precise tools occurred.

All we know is that at some later date the points that up to that time had only been pressed were punctured with needles in order to intensify the healing effect. Special acupuncture needles were developed to penetrate the skin and remain in place for a while. When carried out by an experienced therapist, this procedure is usually painless.

TIP

If you find acupressure techniques helpful, you may want to try acupuncture, too. Although acupuncture is usually painless, it should be administered only by a trained practitioner. Acupuncture is not suitable for self-treatment!

A Word of Caution!

Never try to use acupuncture on yourself. If used incorrectly, acupuncture can lead to serious problems. However, you can safely use acupressure on yourself if you follow a few basic rules.

The Effects of Acupressure

What Exactly Is Acupressure?

We still don't know for certain how acupuncture and acupressure actually work. What we do know, however, is that there is greater skin resistance at the acupuncture points along the meridians. Thus, by measuring this resistance, we can prove the existence of the meridians. The effectiveness of acupressure and acupuncture treatment has been demonstrated in the laboratory by measuring heart reactions.

Stimulating the points with needles or with finger pressure is a painless way of getting the energetic equilibrium back into harmony again.

Acupressure is nothing more than the gentle treatment of the acupuncture points without using needles. Because it is almost impossible to make mistakes when doing this, acupressure is excellent for self-treatment.

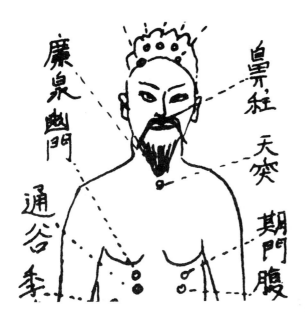

Chinese books hundreds of years ago discussed treatment methods and described the meridians and their acupressure and acupuncture points. Today, we have returned to these ancient methods and find them surprisingly effective.

Complex Benefits

Tests have proved that acupressure and acupuncture stimulate the formation of endomorphines, the body's own "painkillers," which can have the same powerful effect as morphine itself. Acupuncture and acupressure work. They stimulate the nerve fibers, easing the pain and activating the self-healing powers of the body. In other words, they build up energy again in areas where there was a deficit, or they remove an excess of energy.

Acupressure and the Body's Organs

Just as every pressure point relates to a certain meridian or organ, every reflex influences the yin energy and the yang energy of the body. Depending on the direction of the acupressure, you are stimulating or soothing the autonomic nervous system. This balances the energy and restores harmony.

Elaborate testing and measuring methods have proven the positive effects of acupressure. Of course, a simple way of demonstrating the effectiveness is to observe how the patient feels after treatment.

Acupressure

☛ Stimulates the circulatory system, especially the arteries that supply the organs with blood rich in oxygen

☛ Stimulates the function of the hormonal glands

☛ Has a calming and relaxing effect

☛ Is highly suitable for self-treatment

☛ Eases pain by creating the body's "painkillers," the endomorphines

☛ Effectively activates the body's self-healing powers

☛ Ensures drainage of the lymph glands and metabolic wastes

Acupressure Techniques

Different Styles

Over the years, many different techniques of applying acupressure have developed. You will find that every experienced acupressurist has his or her own style. After you have treated yourself for a while, you will discover the technique that works best for you. There are four popular techniques:

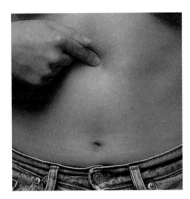

Self-treatment with acupressure.

Tapping

Tap the acupressure points with your index finger.

Pressing

Put the tip of your thumb, your index finger, or your middle finger on the acupressure point, and move it in a circle around the point, while applying firm pressure to the skin.

Effleurage

Slide the tip of your thumb along an acupressure line or zone. This technique is especially useful on large parts of the skin, such as the back.

Wooden Rod Technique

If you want to press very firmly, you can use sticks made of rosewood to apply pressure to the points.

After trying different ones, you will discover which of the four acupressure techniques is best for you.

Techniques for Relaxing or Stimulating

If you want to relax a specific body part, called sedating, your touch should be soothing. You should apply acupressure in a clockwise, circular motion from the inside to the outside.

If you want to stimulate a specific body part, called toning, you should always work in a circular motion counterclockwise, from the outside to the inside.

You will find an R for relaxing (sedating) or an S for stimulating (toning) prior to the optimal treatment times for each common complaint.

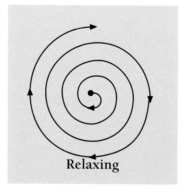

Relaxing

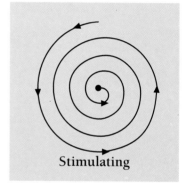

Stimulating

General Guidelines

Every person is different, so acupressure affects everyone differently. Thus, we cannot create an exact program of self-treatment that will be right for each individual.

You can use up to three acupressure treatments a day, depending on the disorder. Each treatment should last from one to 10 minutes. Take more care in treating infants—30 seconds should be sufficient. Generally, you can rely on the reaction of your body. This means that you will feel when it is time to stop.

Allow Time for Improvement

Acupressure has a regulating effect on the autonomic nervous system; therefore, it is especially well suited to treating anxiety, regardless of whether the anxiety is acute or chronic. Be patient during your treatment, and allow three to four weeks before expecting any improvement in your condition.

What You Should Know Before Starting Self-Treatment

You have to be patient. You cannot expect success within a few days, especially when treating nervous disorders. But once you have achieved success, it will be long lasting.

☛ Make sure that you will not be disturbed; disconnect the telephone and, if possible, the doorbell.
☛ Lie down or sit down and relax. Concentrate on the treatment and its effect.
☛ Breathe from the diaphragm. Breathe in through your nose (your abdomen will expand), and hold your breath for a short while. Breathe out (your diaphragm will rise).
☛ Quiet, calming music can be supportive.
☛ Never use self-treatment immediately after taking any kind of painkiller.
☛ Do not drink any alcoholic beverages before treatment.
☛ Do not extend your treatment for more than 25 minutes.
☛ Your hands should be warm, and your fingernails should be short.
☛ Never treat yourself when you are pressed for time; concentrate on the individual skin points.
☛ Stop self-treatment immediately if you experience pain.

☛ With acute complaints, you can treat yourself up to three times daily.

☛ Except for the conception vessel and the governing vessel, the meridians are always found in pairs. Thus, you should treat the points on both sides of the body simultaneously or one side immediately after the other.

☛ For chronic complaints, treat yourself once a day for no longer than 25 minutes.

☛ A partner can work on all acupressure points, especially those on the back that are difficult to reach. Bear in mind that recommendations concerning measurements, such as the width of one finger, always relate to the size of the patient's own body!

☛ All acupressure points mentioned in this book were chosen because they are easy to find and easy to reach for self-treatment.

A partner can help you by massaging the points that are difficult for you to reach. In addition, many people are able to relax easily when they are being treated by someone they know and trust.

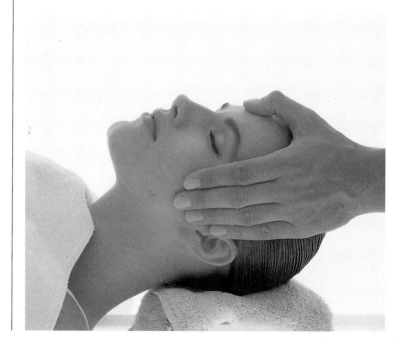

How to Find the Right Pressure Point

You can buy a battery-operated pen that can help you find the point. If you are interested in a simple, less expensive way, remember that the Chinese have not had any technical devices at their disposal during the past 6,000 years. Use the same techniques that they used.

☛ Touch yourself gently around the area on your skin where the point is supposed to be located.

☛ You will find only one spot that is more sensitive than the surrounding skin. With a little experience, you will be able to detect a slight hollow there.

☛ It will be easier for you to find the point again if you mark it with a felt-tip pen.

The Limitations of Acupressure

All advantages have some disadvantages.

☛ Remember that self-treatment can never be a substitute for any treatment or operation that your physician considers necessary.

☛ You should not treat yourself if you suffer from a serious cardiac or circulatory disorder or if you have any severe inflammatory illness.

☛ Do not treat skin areas where there is acne, an allergic skin disorder, discharges of pus, open wounds, or fungal infections (mycosis) because of the danger of infecting another person or of reinfecting yourself.

Be careful when you are unsure of a situation. Certain points should not be treated during pregnancy. In order to avoid dangerous circumstances, consult a physician or a trained acupressurist.

TIP
Forget about expensive electronic devices, and use your own touch to locate the points. You are your own best monitor. In the beginning, after you locate the points, mark them with a felt-tip pen. This will help you find them again later.

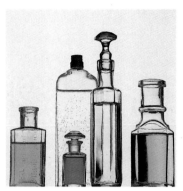

Aromatic oils can be used with acupressure.

The best times for treatment are given with every acupressure description. If the time is especially suitable for relaxing or stimulating, you will find an R or an S in front of it (see page 24).

Treatments for Common Complaints

On the following pages, you will find common complaints listed in alphabetical order with their recommended course of treatment; you can find special recommendations for treating children starting on page 77.

Detailed Drawings to Facilitate the Search for Points

We have included one or more detailed drawings for every complaint. These will show you exactly where to apply treatment. You will find a drawing showing the most important meridians on the inside of the back cover of the book.

If you are not completely sure about an acupressure point, you don't need to rely on the drawing alone; try to feel your way to the point. Very often you will be able to feel when you have reached the right point.

Test: Finding the Pressure Point

As an exercise, try to find pressure-point LI 4. This point, with the poetic name Hegu, "Meeting in the Valley," is so tender that you will get immediate feedback when you have found it.

☛ Press your thumb against your extended index finger. You will notice a slight rise in one of the muscles on the back of your hand.

☛ You will find LI 4 under the highest point of this rise or very close to it.

☛ If you feel around this point, you will notice that it is much more sensitive than the surrounding area.

Aromatherapy as an Adjunct to Acupressure

Sometimes we wouldn't know what we are eating without our sense of smell. Nor would we be aware of the marvelous aroma of a rose or be warned of pungent or corrosive vapors. We react in a very direct and intensive way to what our nose tells us, even though this process takes place subconsciously most of the time.

Our Sense of Smell Helps in Healing

Natural aromatic oils have a medicinal effect. This is the basis of aromatherapy. Aromatic oils come from plants that have specific chemical and physical properties, although further research is needed for us to fully understand the composition of many of these oils. What we do know, however, is that when the aroma of these oils enters the air around us, it is picked up by the mucous membranes of the nose, and it launches its healing effect.

Natural aromatic oils can do the following:

☛ have a stimulating effect on all secreting glands
☛ stimulate the peristaltic muscles
☛ act as a strong disinfectant
☛ act as an antiseptic
☛ have a relaxing and calming effect
☛ have a stimulating and invigorating effect
☛ stimulate both psychologically and autonomically

Many of these oils are very suitable as adjuncts to acupressure treatment. Therefore, we have listed references to appropriate substances for every complaint.

You can inhale the vapors of aromatic oils by using a special scent lamp filled with water, or you can just put a few drops on your pillow at night.

Relaxation is an important prerequisite for success in an acupressure treatment. Therefore, aromatherapy is a very suitable supportive measure.

TIP
Put a drop of the aromatic oil on an acupressure point, and then massage the spot.

TREATMENT

● LI 2—*Erjian*
Large-intestine meridian, point 2
At the second joint of the index finger

● LI 3— *Sonjian*
Large-intestine meridian, point 3
In the small depression at the end of the third joint of the index finger formed when pressing your thumb against your index finger

● LI 4— *Hegu*
Large-intestine meridian, point 4
Press your thumb against your extended index finger, and you will see a bulge in the muscle. The highest point of the bulge is the acupressure point.

● LU 7— *Lieque*
Lung meridian, point 7
In the depression between the ulna and the radius above the wrist

S 5–7 A.M., *7–9* A.M.

Aromatic oil: sage

Acne

This irritating and unattractive skin condition causes a great deal of unhappiness because it seriously affects self-confidence. In some cases, acne is hereditary. It often appears during puberty. Bacteria cause the inflammation of the sebaceous glands and hair follicles, which results in festering pimples. Young people often suffer from acne during puberty because their hormones are not balanced.

When acne occurs after puberty, it is usually due to an imbalance of hormones or a metabolic disorder. Acne also can be caused by eating the wrong foods, a lack of skin hygiene, or serious psychological conflicts.

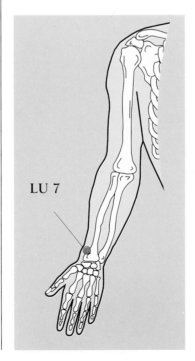
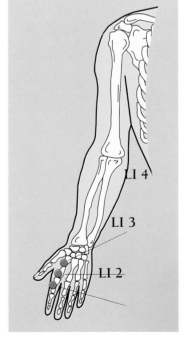

Allergies

More and more people these days are plagued with allergies. Most of them are caused by environmental pollutants that weaken the immune system.

Sometimes a certain area of the skin is affected because it has come in contact with an allergen. Allergins can be found in cosmetics, ointments, medicines, and soaps, or their preserving agents. The food that you eat also can be the cause of an allergic skin reaction. For example, many people are allergic to fresh strawberries. In addition, the causative agents can be substances such as pollen, grasses, certain proteins in foods, or a combination of ingredients in some medicines.

The symptoms usually include a reddening of the skin, which may be accompanied by an itchy or burning sensation.

Acupressure can shorten the healing process. However, if you suffer from an allergy, it is wise to consult a physician.

TREATMENT

● *LI 3— Sonjian*
Large-intestine meridian, point 3
If you spread your fingers, you find this point in the indentation formed between the third joint of the index finger and the thumb.

● *LI 4— Hegu*
Large-intestine meridian, point 4
When you press your thumb and forefinger together, you will find this point on the highest spot of the bulge of the muscle.

● *LU 7— Lieque*
Lung meridian, point 7
In the depression between the ulna and radius

● *LU 9— Taiyuan*
Lung meridian, point 9
At the outer end of the main wrist furrow

3–5 P.M., R 5–7 P.M.

Aromatic oil: chamomile

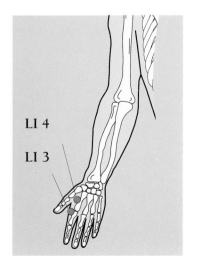

LI 4
LI 3

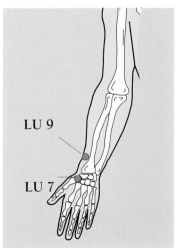

LU 9
LU 7

TREATMENT

● *H 9—Shaochong*
Heart meridian, point 9
The nail wall (perionychium) of
the little finger

● *H 7—Shenmen*
Heart meridian, point 7
Just inside the furrow of the
wrist

● *H 5—Tongli*
Heart meridian, point 5
At the furrow of the wrist, the
width of two fingers above H7
Apply firm pressure on each
point for 1 to 2 minutes.

● *You can also apply gentle*
acupressure to two points on
the ear. Hold your right ear,
and massage each point clock-
wise.

R 11 A.M.–1 P.M.

Aromatic oils: orange blossom,
tangerine

Anxiety

Anxiety is a frequent occurrence. People experience anxiety in different ways with varied intensity. The symptoms can include exhaustion, apathy, restlessness, insomnia, hyperactivity, and aggressiveness. Panic attacks are a form of anxiety. The fear of another attack leads to a vicious cycle. The body reacts with symptoms such as blood-pressure disorders, dizziness, breathing difficulties, or shooting pains and cramps behind the breastbone. Other symptoms may be loss of appetite and diarrhea. Shivering and cold, clammy hands can alternate with excessive perspiration.

It is very important to find out what caused the anxiety in order to come up with an effective treatment. If anxiety remains untreated for long periods of time, it can result in serious physical disorders.

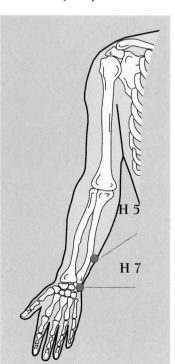

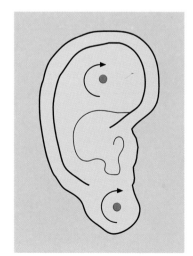

Appetite Problems

Psychological factors such as unhappiness, depression, and anxiety can cause a loss of appetite. However, infections, the common cold, or even an upset stomach also can produce appetite problems. Consult a physician if a loss of appetite continues for more than a few days.

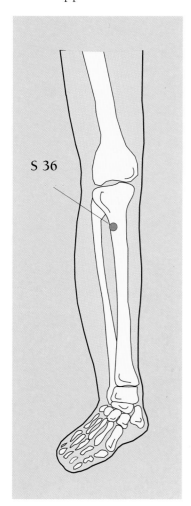

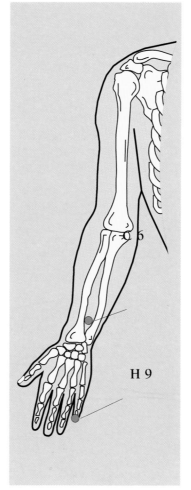

TREATMENT

● *S 36—Zusanli*
Stomach meridian, point 36
Located just below the kneecap on the outside of the shinbone (tibia), this point increases energy in every meridian and is good for the digestion.

● *H 9—Shaochong*
Heart meridian, point 9
On the nail wall of the little finger

● *C 6— Neiguan*
Circulation meridian, point 6
On the middle of the inside of the forearm, the width of three fingers below the bend of the wrist

Treatment should always begin 30 minutes after meals.

1–3, 9–11 P.M., S 9–11 A.M.

Aromatic oil: marjoram

TREATMENT

Arthritis

Pains in the Knee
● *S 35—Dubi*
Stomach meridian, point 35
On the outside of the knee joint

● *S 36—Zusanli*
Stomach meridian, point 15
The outside of the shinbone (tibia)

Pains in the Shoulder
● *LI 15—Jianyu*
Large-intestine meridian, point 15
The outside of the shoulder

● *SI 11—Tianzong*
Small-intestine meridian, point 11
Where the spinal process joins the fourth spinal vertebra on the shoulder

R 5–7 A.M., 7–9 A.M., 1–3 P.M.

Aromatic oils: juniper, eucalyptus

Arthritis is an acute or chronic inflammation of one or more joints. It is a degenerative disease. Osteoarthritis is a form of arthritis in which the cartilage between the bones disintegrates, and the surfaces of the two bones rub directly against each other. The result is severe pain and stiffness in the affected joint.

Acupressure is able to counteract the pain and the restricted movement, and to help slow down the degenerative process.

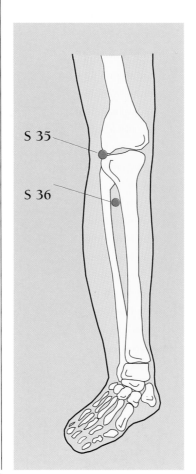

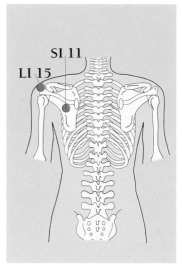

Asthma

Breathing difficulties are an indication that someone or something is interfering with our freedom and independence, and we can no longer breathe freely. We will not be able to breathe freely again until we resolve the problems or solve the difficulty.

A person who is suffering from asthma has a disturbance in the balance between giving and taking, and all too often, someone is taking too much. The bronchial tubes become cramped, and the air overexpands the lungs. This leads to the typical symptoms of asthma. On the other hand, we may be too interested in material things or put too much emphasis on emotions, attention, and love without reciprocating to those around us. The next stage is the withdrawal stage; we block off everything coming from the outside. Thus, anxiety sets up a protective reflex action in the diaphragm.

Those suffering from asthma will find it helpful to face their anxieties and repressed aggressions and start talking about their problems. This can help an asthmatic accept love and give it as well.

TREATMENT

● *LI 4—Hegu*
Large-intestine meridian, point 4
Press your thumb against your extended index finger, and you will see a bulge in the muscle. The highest point of the bulge is the acupressure point.

● *LU 6—Kongzui*
Lung meridian, point 6
On the inside of the forearm, the width of seven fingers above the bend of the wrist

● *LU 7—Lieque*
Lung meridian, point 7
In the hollow between the ulna and radius above the wrist

● *C 6 —Neiguan*
Circulation meridian, point 6
On the inside of the middle of the forearm, the width of three fingers below the bend of the wrist

R 3 – 5 A.M., 7 – 9 P.M.

Aromatic oil: sandalwood

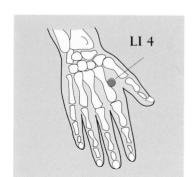

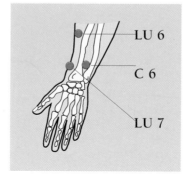

Backache

Many adults and an increasing number of young people suffer from backaches. Backaches can be due to a simple weakness, a degeneration of the spine, rheumatic disorders (see page 68), or a slipped disk (see page 71).

The main causes, however, are lack of exercise and incorrect posture. If you do not exercise and you spend the entire day in your office sitting in an unsuitable chair, you should not be surprised if your back starts to act up.

Psychological problems also can have a direct effect on the back. Observe yourself and your posture in order to discover if you are letting your problems wear you down or if you are overstressed.

TREATMENT

● *GV 2—Yaoshu*
Governing vessel, point 2
At the end of the buttocks fold, between the coccyx and the sacrum

● *B 31—Shangliao*
Bladder meridian, point 31
In the hollow of the sacrum

R 3–5 P.M.

Aromatic oil: sandalwood

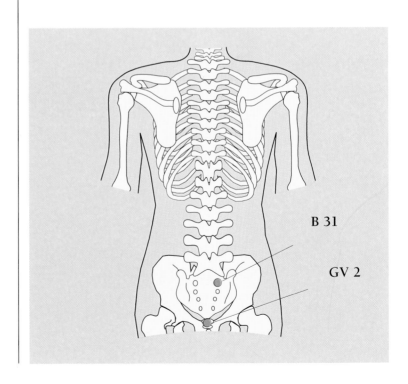

B 31

GV 2

Belching and Heartburn

Fermentation in the intestines and hyperacidity in the stomach can cause these problems. Foods such as radishes and cabbage also can be the culprit because of their composition.

Swallowing too much air often causes children to belch.

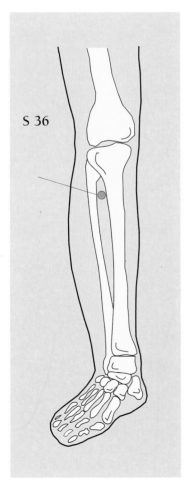
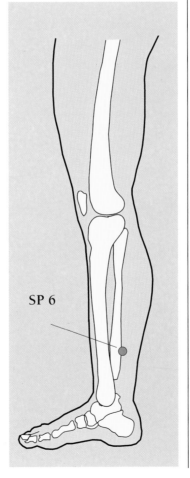

TREATMENT

● *S 36—Zusanli*
Stomach meridian, point 36
The width of one finger to the side of the shinbone (tibia)

R 7–9 A.M.

● *SP 6—Sanyinjiao*
Spleen-pancreas meridian, point 6
Behind the shinbone (tibia)

R 9–11 A.M.

Aromatic oil: peppermint

TREATMENT

● *H 7—Shenmen*
Heart meridian, point 7
In the bend of the wrist

● *H 3—Shaohai*
Heart meridian, point 3
At the end of the bend of the elbow

● *LI 4—Hegu*
Large-intestine meridian, point 4
Press your thumb against your extended index finger, and you will see a bulge in the muscle. The highest point of the bulge is the acupressure point.

7–9 A.M., S 1–3 P.M.

Aromatic oil: rosemary

Blood Pressure, Low

When you have low blood pressure, you usually feel the effects in the morning. You feel dizzy when you get up too quickly, you are tired, and you need a good deal of time to get started with your morning routine. In addition, fainting is fairly common in the morning or at any time during the day .

People who suffer from low blood pressure often give in to their problems, and then they feel depressed. When they have to face a problem with which they cannot cope, they often feel helpless and weak.

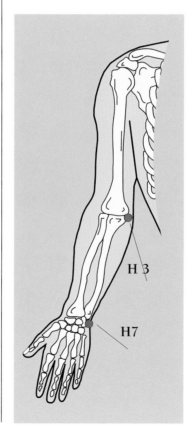

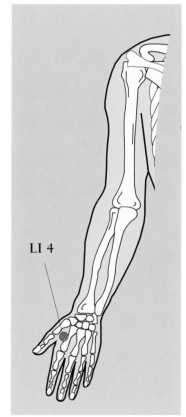

Breathing Difficulties

It's important to differentiate between temporary breathing difficulties, which can be caused by having a cold or by cigarette or cigar smoke, and true shortness of breath. If the latter occurs when you are climbing stairs, for instance, it is usually an indication of some heart or circulatory disorder, and you must see a specialist for treatment. According to the "language of our organs," breath is a symbol of life, so if you have difficulties breathing you have to ask yourself: "What is it that is making it so hard for me to breathe?" Breathing difficulties are often due to some psychological factor.

TREATMENT

● *LI 4—Hegu*
Large-intestine meridian, point 4
Press your thumb against your extended index finger, and you will see a bulge in the muscle. The highest point of the bulge is the acupressure point.

● *C 6—Neiguan*
Circulation meridian, point 6
In the middle of the inside of the forearm, the width of three fingers below the bend of the wrist

● *LU 5—Chize*
Lung meridian, point 5
In the middle of the bend of the elbow

3–5 A.M., R 5–7 A.M., 7–9 P.M.

Aromatic oil: eucalyptus

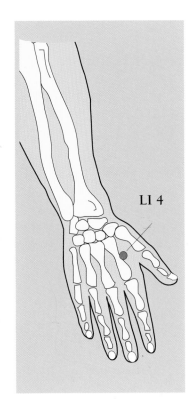

LI 4

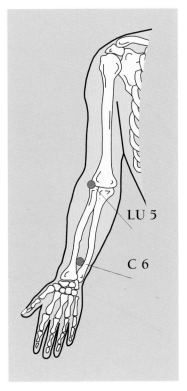

LU 5

C 6

Bronchitis

Bronchitis is often caused by influenza. Other possible culprits are cold weather conditions, dust, and cigarette smoke. Bronchitis is an acute inflammation of the bronchial tubes. It is accompanied by a painful, dry cough at the beginning. After a while, the patient starts to cough up phlegm. If the coughing becomes painful or if the sputum is a yellowish green or contains blood, the patient should see a physician immediately. These acupressure points will loosen the phlegm so that it can be coughed up.

TREATMENT

● *LU 1— Zhonfu*
Lung meridian, point 1
Between the first and second ribs

● *LU 5—Chize*
Lung meridian, point 9
At the middle of the bend of the elbow

● *LU 9—Taiyuan*
Lung meridian, point 9
At the outer end of the bend of the wrist

R 3–5 A.M.

Aromatic oil:eucalyptus

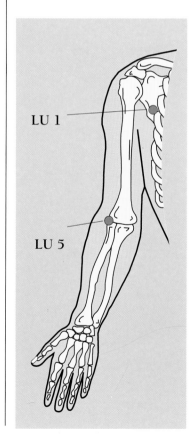
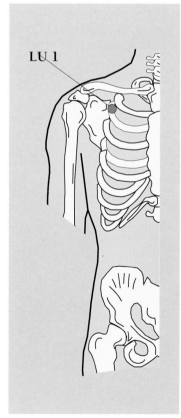

Colds

Colds often keep us at home, flat on our back in bed. The average adult has two to four colds a year; the average for children is higher. We are all familiar with the symptoms of a runny nose, hoarseness, sore throat, aching joints, and fatigue. These range from mild to severe. Regardless of the severity of the symptoms, the body is saying that it is busy fighting germs and needs extra rest and special care for a while.

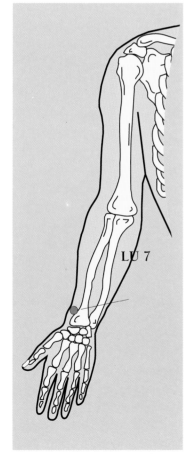

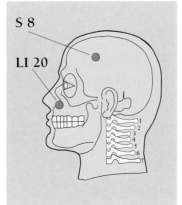

TREATMENT

● *LI 20—Yingxiang*
Large-intestine meridian, point 20
On the lateral fold between the nose and upper lip

● *S 8—Touwei*
Stomach meridian, point 8
At the hairline, just above the temple

● *LU 5—Chize*
Lung meridian, point 5
In the middle of the bend of the elbow

● *LU 7—Lieque*
Lung meridian, point 7
In the furrow between the ulna and radius above the wrist

R 5–7 A.M., *S 7–9* A.M., *9–11* A.M.

Aromatic oils: eucalyptus, sage

TREATMENT

● *LI 4 Hegu*
Large-intestine meridian, point 4
Press your thumb against your extended index finger, and you will see a bulge in the muscle. The highest point of the bulge is the acupressure point.

● *LI 10—Shousanli*
Large-intestine meridian, point 10
On the outside of the lower arm

● *LI 11—Quchi*
Large-intestine meridian, point 11
At the very end of the elbow furrow

● *S 36—Zusanli*
Stomach meridian, point 36
On the outside of the shinbone (tibia)

S 7–9 A.M., 9–11 A.M.

Aromatic oil: peppermint

Constipation

Frequently a lifestyle consisting of too much sitting and too little exercise is the cause of constipation (see Intestinal Disorders, page 54). In addition, your diet may not be supplying your digestive system with enough fiber. Dietary fiber stimulates the intestines, ensuring that they work properly. You need a balanced diet and plenty of exercise to help your intestines do their job. Acupressure helps you stimulate the intestines even more.

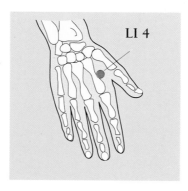

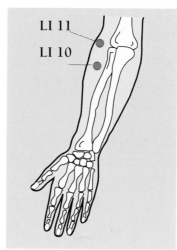

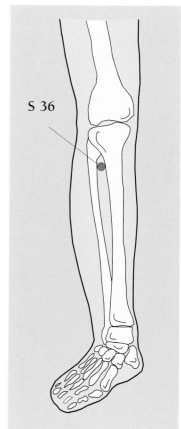

Coughing

When you cough, your body is trying to clear the respiratory tract so that you can breathe freely. Any irritation or inflammation of the respiratory system causes you to cough in order to get rid of the phlegm, dust, and so forth. If coughing continues for more than three weeks, you should consult your physician.

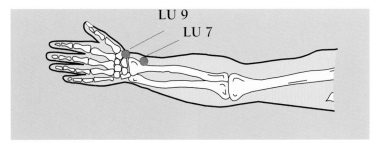

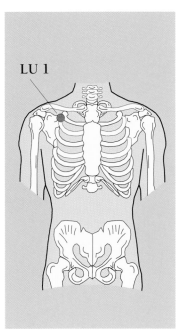

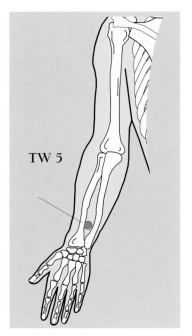

TREATMENT

● *LU 1—Zhongfu*
Lung meridian, point 1
Between the first and second ribs

● *TW 5—Waiguan*
Triple-warmer meridian, point 5
On the back of the lower arm

● *LU 7—Lieque*
Lung meridian, point 7
In the hollow between the ulna and radius above the wrist

● *LU 9—Taiyuan*
Lung meridian, point 9
At the outer end of the bend of the wrist

R 3–5 A.M., *9–11* P.M.

Aromatic oil: sage

TREATMENT

● *H 3— Shaohai*
Heart meridian, point 3
At the outer end of the bend in
the elbow

● *H 7—Shenmen*
Heart meridian, point 7
The inner end of the bend of the
wrist

● *S 36—Zusanli*
Stomach meridian, point 36
On the outer side of the shin-
bone (tibia)

● *S 41—Jiexi*
Stomach meridian, point 41
In the middle of the tarsal
bones

S 1–3 P.M., *9–11* A.M.

Aromatic oil: orange blossom

Depression

Depression is often an expression of deep psychological pain. It also may be the result of shock and the suppressed aggressions one has after shock. Bottled-up emotions can cause lasting feelings of despondency. People often need to talk about such problems with an experienced therapist in order to improve.

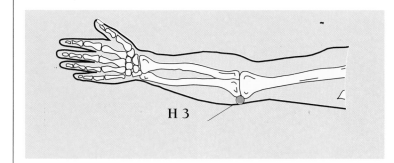

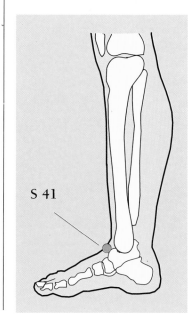

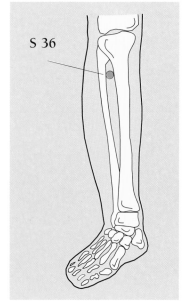

Diarrhea

This unpleasant and often painful disorder of the intestines can have many causes: spoiled food, infections, intestinal flu, certain medicines, metabolic ailments, and even excitement and stress (see Intestinal Disorders, page 54). If diarrhea continues for more than three days, consult your physician, because the loss of body fluids can result in an imbalance of acids and bases in your system.

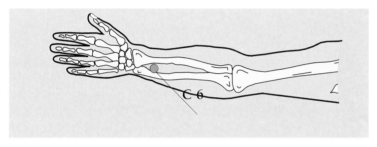

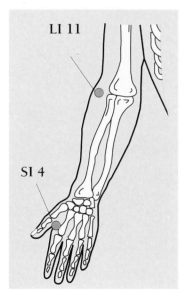

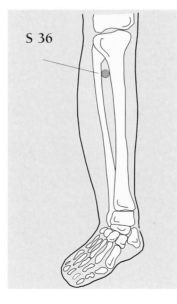

TREATMENT

● *S 36— Zusanli*
Stomach meridian, point 36
On the outside of the shinbone (tibia)

● *SI 4— Hegu*
Small-intestine meridian, point 4
Press your thumb against your extended index finger, and you will see a bulge in the muscle. The highest point of the bulge is the acupressure point.

● *LI 11—Quchi*
Large-intestine Meridian, point 11
At the outer end of the bend in the elbow

● *C 6—Neiguan*
Circulation meridian, point 6
In the middle of the inside of the forearm, the width of three fingers below the bend of the wrist

5–7 A.M., R 7–9 A.M., 7–9 P.M.

Aromatic oil: geranium

Eyelids, Swollen

Swollen eyes and lachrymal sacs are irritating and unattractive. Given time, they usually disappear by themselves without treatment. However, if they remain swollen, the lymphs may not be draining properly, and the venous pressure may be increasing.

This can be the result of a hormonal problem, but it also may be a sign of a kidney or bladder disorder. You should consult a specialist if the edema does not go away. It also is possible that your blood pressure is dropping considerably at night when you are lying down, and, as a result, your eyes are swollen the next morning.

People who suffer from frequent or chronic eyelid edema and swollen lachrymal sacs usually do not want to face their problems, or they want to shut their eyes rather than deal with their problems.

However, if the edema is just a result of fatigue, stress, too much alcohol, or a similar problem, acupressure can make the swelling go down quickly.

TREATMENT

● *TW 5—Waiguan*
Triple-warmer meridian, point 5
On the back of the lower arm

S 11 P.M.–1 A.M

Aromatic oils are not recommended for this ailment; instead, apply cold compresses with a solution of eyebright or linden blossoms.

TW 5

Fatigue

Fatigue can indicate a lack of minerals such as iron. If you are fatigued regularly, you should consult your physician. Fatigue can be caused by strain or exhaustion, and it also can be a symptom of illness. In the latter case, especially with infection, fatigue occurs when the defense mechanisms of the body are active. Your immune system needs all the strength it can get, so be sure to get enough sleep.

TREATMENT

● SP 2—Dadu
Spleen-pancreas meridian, point 2
At the basal joint of the big toe on the inside of the foot

● SP 5—Shangqui
Spleen-pancreas meridian, point 5
Above the ankle joint

● G 24—Riyue
Gallbladder meridian, point 24
Between the fifth and sixth ribs

● GV 19—Houding
Governing vessel, point 19
On the posterior fontanel at the back of the head

S 11 A.M.–1 P.M., 1–3 P.M.

Aromatic oil: peppermint

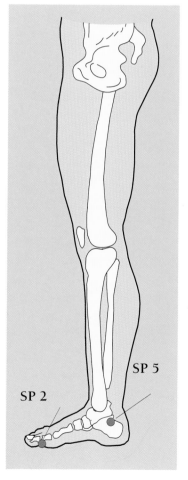

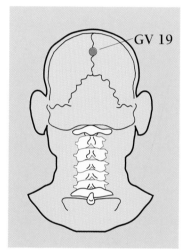

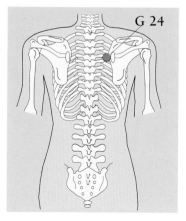

TREATMENT

● *SP 2—Dadu*
Spleen-pancreas meridian,
point 2
In the middle of the basal joint
of the big toe

● *SP 5 —Shangqui*
Spleen-pancreas meridian,
point 5
Just below the ankle

● *SP 6— Sanyinjiao*
Spleen-pancreas meridian,
point 6
The width of three fingers
above the ankle

S 11 A.M.*–1* P.M.

Aromatic oils: peppermint,
eucalyptus

Feet, Cold

Women often suffer from cold feet. The cause can be low blood pressure or a disturbance in the circulation of the blood in the legs. Sometimes exercise can help: a short walk, some aerobics, and so forth. In addition to being unpleasant and uncomfortable, cold feet can become a health problem. When the extremities are cold, the body reacts by heating the more important areas. Simply put, the body saves energy on the outside in order to have enough energy for the vital inner parts.

However, this lowers the temperature of the mucous membranes as well. The lower temperature of the mucous membranes makes it easier for viruses that cannot live in high temperatures to attack the body. This increases the incidence of colds, the flu, and other problems. The urethra is especially sensitive in such situations. Nearly every woman who suffers from cold feet is also familiar with painful bladder infections.

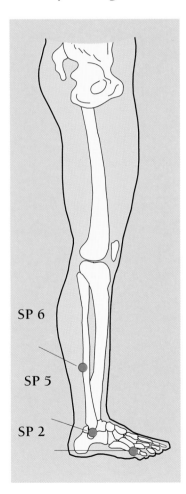

SP 6

SP 5

SP 2

Gallbladder Problems

The gallbladder is the organ that stores the bile produced by the liver. It is very sensitive to an improper diet or psychological disharmony, which may result in gallstones. Gallbladder complaints often plague people who are unable to speak about their hostilities openly and overcome them. Thus, they turn their hostility against themselves in a self-destructive way. In the beginning, gallstones usually do not cause any problems; therefore, they often are not noticed until there is a serious problem. Then, they cause pain in the upper-right side of the abdomen. This pain can extend as far as the right shoulder and into the back. Very severe cases can lead to a gallstone attack with violent pains, vomiting, and a swollen abdomen. When this occurs, you should see your physician immediately. Inflammations of the gallbladder or of the bile duct also must be treated by a physician.

Acupressure helps support the smooth functioning of this important organ. If you tend to have problems with your gallbladder, you should avoid fatty foods.

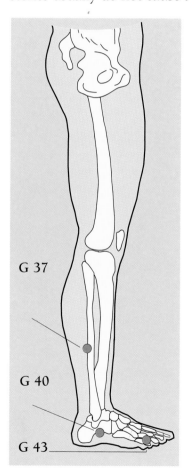

G 37

G 40

G 43

TREATMENT

● G 37—*Guangming*
Gallbladder meridian, point 37
On the outside of the lower leg, just above the ankle

● G 38—*Yangfu*
Gallbladder meridian, point 38
On the outside of the lower leg, next to the edge of the shinbone (tibia)

● G 40—*Qiuxu*
Gallbladder meridian, point 40
On the instep of the foot

● G 43—*Xiaxi*
Gallbladder meridian, point 43
On the outside of the basal joint of the fourth toe

R 11 P.M.–2 A.M.

Aromatic oil: grapefruit

Hair Loss

A loss of hair can occur in a limited area, for example, at the hairline around the temples or in a circular area at the back of the head. However, a slow loss of hair over the entire head is also common. The hair loss can be the result of a functional disorder or the destruction of hair follicles. This can be an inherited problem (many men are affected in this way) or caused by an infection, toxic substances in the body, certain medicines, or hormonal changes. In addition, a fungal infection (mycosis) or stress can bring about hair loss.

TREATMENT

● B 54—Zhibian
Bladder meridian, point 54
In the middle of the hollow of the knee

● S 39—Xiajuxu
Stomach meridian, point 39
The width of six fingers below S 36

9–11 A.M., S 5–7 P.M.

Aromatic oil: rosemary

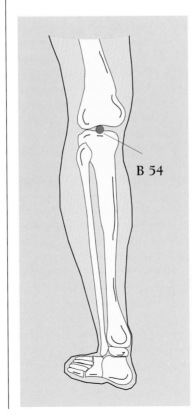

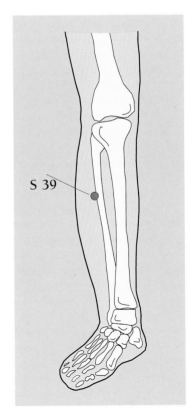

Headaches

Headaches have many different causes and just as many different kinds of pain. The most common pain occurs in conjunction with the outbreak of a cold, with stress, and with certain nervous conditions. Other triggers for headaches can be anxiety, stale air, changes in the weather, and allergic reactions. Women frequently suffer from headaches during menstruation.

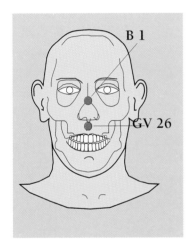

You can obtain quick relief by taking a variety of pills, but a much gentler way is through acupressure. If you have frequent or regular headaches, you should consult your physician in order to rule out any physical disorders before you start self-treatment. Also, pay attention to whether or not you get a headache after extended sunbathing, because this could be a sign of heatstroke.

In addition to acupressure, bathing your arms in cold water is helpful (immerse your arms up to the elbow in cold water for about 30 seconds). Steam baths with herbs or aromatic oils may give you relief as well.

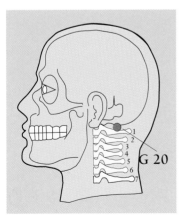

TREATMENT

● *B 1—Jingming*
Bladder meridian, point 1
In the bend at the root of the nose

● *G 20—Fengchi*
Gallbladder meridian, point 20
At the back of the head

● *GV 26—Shuigou*
Governing vessel, point 26
In the middle of the small hollow on the upper lip

R 3–5 P.M., 11 P.M.–1 A.M.

Aromatic oils: orange blossom, lemon balm

TREATMENT

● *TW 6—Zhigou*
Triple-warmer meridian, point 6
The width of three fingers above the skin fold on the back of the wrist

● *LU 6—Kongzui*
Lung meridian, point 6
The width of seven fingers above the fold of the wrist

R 9–11 P.M., 3–5 A.M.

Aromatic oil: chamomile

Hemorrhoids

Although this ailment affects many people, it's only talked about in whispers. Hemorrhoids are a very delicate and painful subject. In most cases, they are caused by a genetic weakness in connective tissue. Because chronic constipation and sitting for long periods of time also can contribute to the development of hemorrhoids, they are sometimes called the "adornment of scholars." People who often are exposed to the cold frequently suffer from hemorrhoids as well. The best prevention is to have enough roughage in your diet and get plenty of exercise.

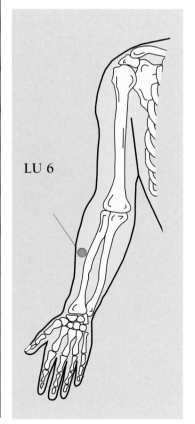

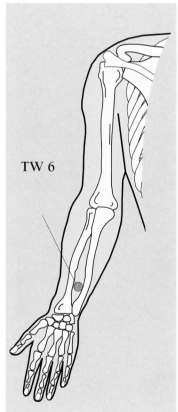

Impotence

TREATMENT

Impotence is usually the result of psychological conflicts having to do with overwork, stress, fear of failure, or sexual pressure. However, it may be wise to consult a specialist before beginning acupressure in order to eliminate any possibility of a physical cause.

● *S 36—Zusanli*
Stomach meridian, point 36
On the outside of the shinbone (tibia)

● *K 3—Taixi*
Kidney meridian, point 3
Between the top of the ankle bone and the Achilles tendon

● *CV 4—Guanyuan*
Conception vessel, point 4
Just above the pubic bone

R 7–9 A.M., 5–6 P.M.

Aromatic oil: ylang-ylang

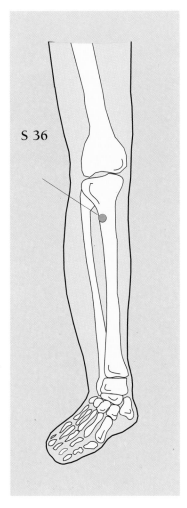

S 36

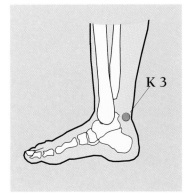

K 3

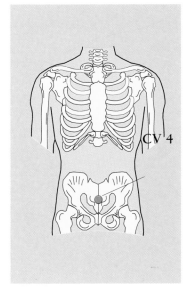

CV 4

TREATMENT

● *SI 3—Houxi*
Small-intestine meridian, point 3
When you make a fist, you will find this point in the fold of the skin on the basal joint of the little finger.

● *SI 8—Xiaohai*
Small-intestine meridian, point 8
The elbow joint

Constipation
3–5 P.M.

Aromatic oil: geranium

Diarrhea
1–3 P.M.

Aromatic oil: peppermint

Intestinal Disorders

The intestines break down and digest everything we eat. The usable substances are separated from the unusable ones. Intestinal disorders often are caused by conflicts and problems that we do not or cannot articulate. Suppressed rage and feelings of hatred, worry, and anxiety all end up in the stomach, leading to intestinal disorders such as constipation and diarrhea.

If we suffer from constipation, the likely problem is that we are not able to let go of a person or a situation. The bowel movement is connected to "giving," and a person who does not want to give may be stingy or trying to hang on to money and other material things.

With diarrhea, the digestive system is working too rapidly. What we take into our body (and mind) leaves in an undigested state (see Diarrhea, page 45).

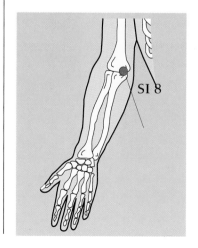

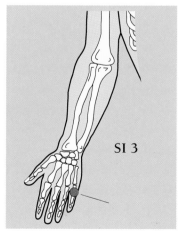

Joint Pains

Problems with the joints can be very painful and produce stiffness. Joint problems have nothing to do with the age of the patient and can even affect young people. Pain in the joints can be the result of injuries, inflammation, pulled ligaments, and sprains. The "language of the organs" defines pain in the joints as stubbornness or defiance on the part of the patient. To alleviate pain in the joints, it helps to get rid of your rigidity and other negative habits.

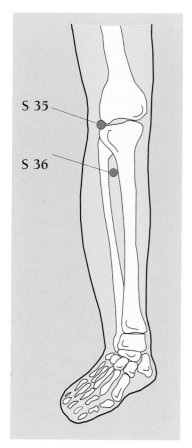

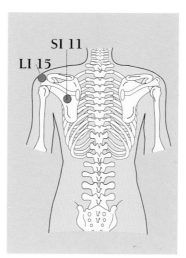

TREATMENT

Knee Problems

● S 35—Dubi
Stomach meridian, point 35
On the outside of the knee joint

● S 36—Zusanli
Stomach meridian, point 36
On the outside of the shinbone (tibia)

Pains in the Shoulder

● LI 15—Jianyu
Large-intestine meridian, point 15
On the outside edge of the shoulder

● SI 11—Tianzong
Small-intestine meridian, point 11
On the shoulder, level with the spinal process of the fourth thoracic vertebra

R 5–7 A.M., 7–9 A.M., 1–3 P.M.

Aromatic oils: juniper, eucalyptus

TREATMENT

● *TW 5—Waiguan*
Triple-warmer meridian, point 5
On the back of the forearm

● *B 58—Feiyang*
Bladder meridian, point 58
On the back of the calf

● *G 40—Qiuxu*
Gallbladder meridian, point 40
On the side of the back of the foot

● *K 2—Xingjiang*
Kidney meridian, point 2
On the basal joint of the big toe

R 3–5 P.M., 11 P.M–1 A.M., 1–3 A.M., 9–11 P.M.

Aromatic oil: rosemary

Leg Cramps

Cramps in the calf muscles of the leg usually occur during the night. The cause is often a disorder of the veins or arteries, or a bone defect such as a deformity of the foot. Disorders of the spine, such as lumbago or slipped disks, or neurological factors also can lead to cramps in the calf muscles. Another culprit could be a low level of potassium, calcium, or magnesium in the blood.

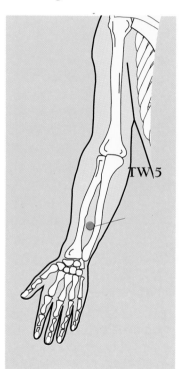

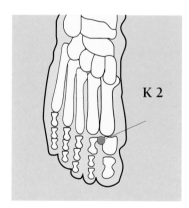

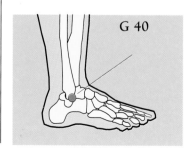

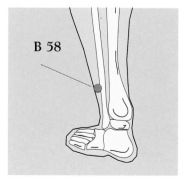

Lumbago

The symptoms of lumbago, a form of rheumatism, are violent pains that hit without warning and a restricted ability to move.

Lumbago can occur when you move abruptly or when you lift or carry heavy objects improperly. Its underlying causes, however, are more complex, and may have to do with incorrect posture that comes from years of too little exercise and sitting incorrectly, or weak back muscles. They affect the body in such a way that the slightest wrong movement, or even cold air blowing on your back, can result in lumbago.

Most of the time, the problem lies in a blockage of the vertebral joints or a slight dislocation of two vertebrae. This causes a painful irritation of the nerve roots.

The best remedies are warm and relaxing baths, liniment, rest, and proper chiropractic treatment (see Slipped Disk, page 71). During the acute stage, lumbago may require bed rest. An orthopedic neck brace is sometimes recommended for lumbago in the neck vertebrae.

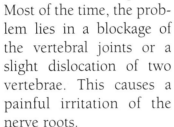
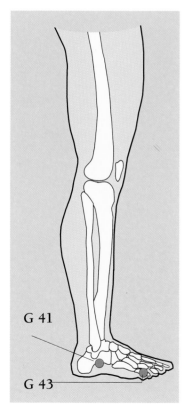

G 41

G 43

TREATMENT

● *G 41—Zulinqui*
Gallbladder meridian, point 41
On the instep of the foot

● *G 43—Xiaxi*
Gallbladder meridian, point 43
On the outside of the basal joint of the fourth toe

R 11 P.M.—1 A.M.

Aromatic oils: rosemary, tea tree

TREATMENT

● B 31—*Shangliao*
Bladder meridian, point 31
In the hollow of the sacrum

● TW 22—*Erheliao*
Triple-warmer meridian, point 22
Above the cheekbone

● SP 6—*Sanyinjiao*
Spleen-pancreas meridian, point 6
On the inside, between the shinbone (tibia) and ankle

9–11 A.M., R 3–5 P.M., 9–11 P.M.

Aromatic oils: orange blossom, geranium

Menopause

During menopause, a woman's body goes through extreme hormonal changes that are comparable to the changes of puberty. The accompanying effects are similar to those of menstruation—pains in the abdomen and the joints, exhaustion, depression, nervousness, and headaches—as well as hot flashes and excessive perspiration. A woman who has difficulty accepting her feminine role—although exactly what that may be is still open to debate—often has more problems with menopause than other women.

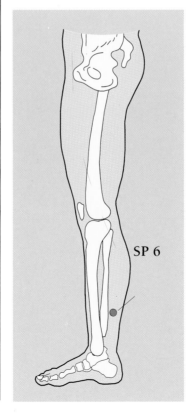

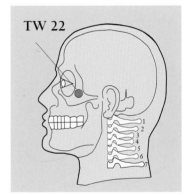

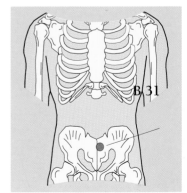

Menstrual Problems

Nearly every women has menstrual problems at one time or another. These may include headaches, stomachaches, backaches, and fatigue, as well as feelings of depression or aggression. The primary reason for all of these problems is a slight disruption in hormonal balance. However, these problems should not be confused with those that occur before menstruation, which we call premenstrual syndrome, or PMS (see page 66).

In the "language of the organs," the different kinds of menstrual problems occur most frequently when women reject their own femininity, although what constitutes femininity is still an issue open to debate. In addition, many women constantly overtax their body, thus creating another basis for menstrual problems.

TREATMENT

● *CV 4—Guanyuan*
Conception vessel, point 4
Above the pubic bone

● *SP 1—Yinbai*
Spleen-pancreas meridian, point 1
In the corner of the big toenail, on the inside of the foot

● *SP 4—Gongsun*
Spleen-pancreas meridian, point 4
In the middle of the inside of the foot

R 9–11 A.M.

Aromatic oils: juniper, rosewood

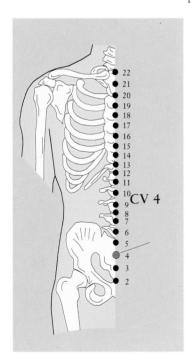

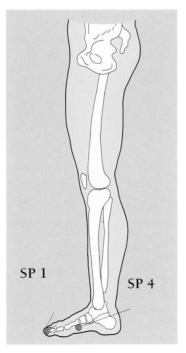

Migraines

Migraine headaches are convulsive, severe headaches often accompanied by spots in front of the eyes, distorted vision, impaired balance, diarrhea, nausea, and vomiting.

Medical researchers have not yet been able to explain the exact cause of the severe pain. However, it is believed that the predisposition to migraines is hereditary. Various factors can trigger a migraine, such as stress (and even a sudden period of rest after stress), certain types of light or odors, some foods, and certain hormonal factors (especially for women). Psychological causes include self-punishment, unfulfilled sexuality, and some kinds of anxiety.

Consult your physician should the pain become unbearable, necessitating strong medication.

TREATMENT

● *CV 12—Zhongwan*
Conception vessel, point 12
The width of four fingers above the navel

● *SP 21—Dabao*
Spleen-pancreas meridian, point 21
Between the ribs

● *GV 12—Shenzu*
Governing vessel, point 12
On the spinal process of the third thoracic vertebra

R 9–11 A.M.

Aromatic oil: marjoram

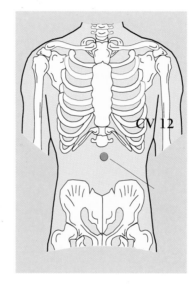

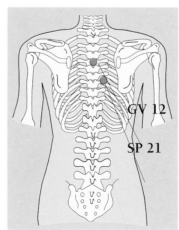

Motion Sickness

What we call motion sickness, including seasickness, occurs because of a communication problem between the vestibular system of the ear and the brain. This can bring on severe nausea and vomiting.

An easy way to prevent motion sickness is to look at an object in the distance. If you are traveling by car, you should fix your eyes on the mountains or anything in the distance; on an ocean voyage, you should watch the horizon. If you read in a moving vehicle, your sense of balance registers the movement, and this conflicts with your sense of vision, which is concentrating on a fixed point. The simple solution is not to read when you are moving. In addition, be sure that you have plenty of fresh air and use the acupressure points recommended here.

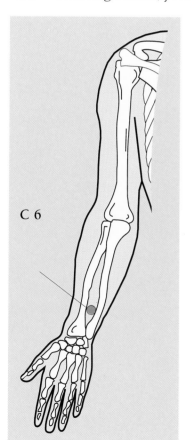

C 6

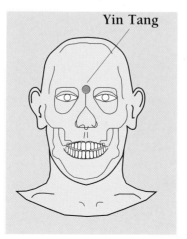

Yin Tang

TREATMENT

● *C 6—Neiguan*
Circulation meridian, point 6
On the middle of the inside of the lower arm, the width of three fingers above the bend of the wrist

● *Yin Tang*
Between the eyebrows

R 7–9 P.M.

Aromatic oil: chamomile

TREATMENT

● *H 7— Shenmen*
Heart meridian, point 7
In the bend of the wrist

● *B 60—Kunlun*
Bladder meridian, point 60
On the outside of the heel

● *B 62— Shenmai*
Bladder meridian, point 62
The width of two fingers below
the ankle

R 11 A.M.*–1* P.M., *3–5* P.M.

Aromatic oil: sandalwood

Nervousness

Many people suffer from nervousness. It even affects children. Nervousness is caused by a malfunctioning of the central nervous system. This happens when you are constantly subjected to external stimuli, overtaxing your system.

The following symptoms often accompany nervousness: insomnia, heart palpitations, excessive perspiration, and anxiety.

If the condition is acute, acupressure can help you relax quickly. For a lasting effect, however, you will have to change your way of living. Try to reduce stress in your job. In your spare time, do exercises that increase your stamina without the pressure of having to succeed. You also can read books instead of switching from one TV channel to another. In addition, yoga or meditation can help you feel calmer and more balanced.

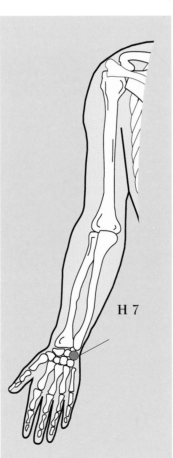

H 7

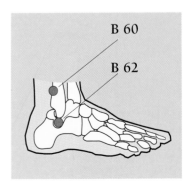

B 60

B 62

Obesity

Obesity is usually due to an improper psychological attitude toward food and eating. To start with, you must discover the reasons why you eat too much or why the food you eat turns into fat too quickly.

A balanced diet, lots of exercise, and fresh air help your body burn food faster, and, at the same time, they make you feel better physically and more stable psychologically. If you like your body, you will hardly ever put on too much weight. If you are overeating because of stress, relaxation techniques such as yoga or meditation will be of help, in addition to acupressure.

TREATMENT

● *TW 3—Zhongzu*
Triple-warmer meridian, point 3
On the basal joint of the ring finger

● *CV 12—Zhongwan*
Conception vessel, point 12
The width of four fingers above the navel

● *S 36—Zusanli*
Stomach meridian, point 36
On the outside of the shinbone (tibia)

S 11 P.M.–1 A.M., 9–11 A.M.

Aromatic oil: juniper

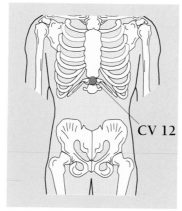

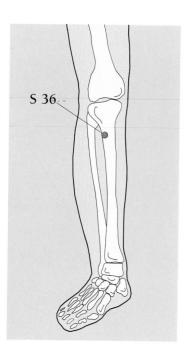

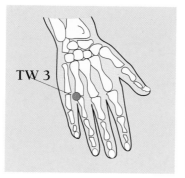

Pregnancy

Today, most women plan their pregnancies very carefully, leaving nothing to chance. They have a positive attitude toward their body. They take care of themselves, especially during pregnancy, and this includes eating a balanced diet.

Their strong frame of mind and their positive attitude allow them to be very receptive to natural methods of healing. That is why pregnant women are able

TREATMENT

Sickness and Vomiting During Pregnancy

● *CV 12—Zhongwan*
Conception vessel, point 12
The width of four fingers above the navel

● *CV 6 —Neiguan*
Conception vessel, point 6
On the inside of the forearm, the width of three fingers above the bend of the wrist

● *S 36—Zusanli*
Stomach meridian, point 36
On the outside of the shinbone (tibia)

7–9 A.M., *R 7–9* P.M.

Aromatic oil: rosewood

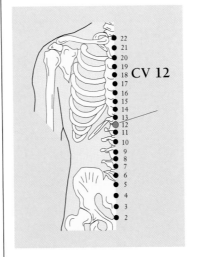

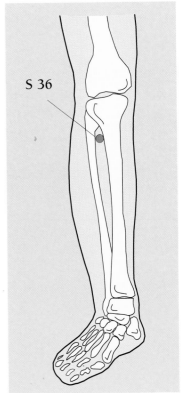

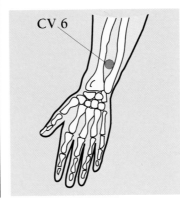

to deal well with acupressure when health problems arise during this time.

Some woman experience feelings of anxiety and uncertainty during pregnancy, so point H 5 (Tongli) is especially effective (see Anxiety, page 32).

Allowing your partner to apply acupressure is best when you are pregnant.

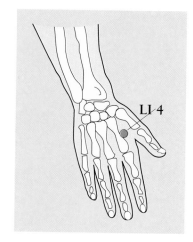

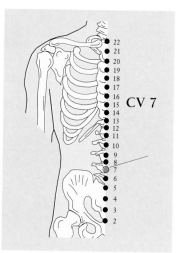

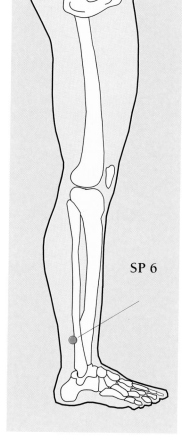

Induction of Labor
● *LI 4— Hegu*
See below.

● *SP 6—Sanyinjiao*
Spleen-pancreas meridian, point 6
The width of three fingers above the ankle

S 7–9 A.M., 11 A.M .–1 P.M.

Aromatic oil: rosemary

Afterpains
● *LI 4—Hegu*
Large-intestine meridian, point 4
Press your thumb against your extended index finger, and you will see a bulge in the muscle. The highest point of the bulge is the acupressure point.

● *CV 7—Yinjiao*
Conception vessel, point 7
The width of one finger below the navel

R 5–7 A.M.

Aromatic oil: balm

65

Premenstrual Syndrome (PMS)

Women often suffer from bloating, stomach cramps, and back pains during the days just before their monthly period. Other symptoms are headaches, which can be migraine in extreme cases, melancholy, hunger, and a craving for sweets, as well as depression or aggression.

All of these symptoms are the result of hormonal changes combined with a lack of vitamin B.

It is important to try to track down the exact causes of these complaints, but acupressure can help to ease the symptoms.

TREATMENT

● CV 3—Zhongji
Conception vessel, point 3
On a line between the pubic bone and the navel

● K 8 —Jiaoxin
Kidney meridian, point 8
On the lower calf, the width of three fingers above the inside of the ankle

● B 31—Shangliao
Bladder meridian, point 31
In the hollow of the sacrum

R 3–5 P.M., 5–6 P.M.

Aromatic oil: sage

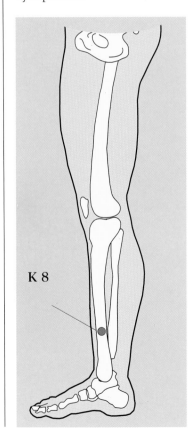

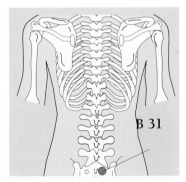

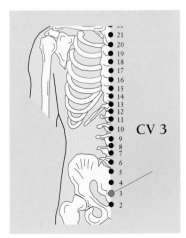

Psoriasis

Psoriasis is a skin disorder and is hereditary. It is triggered by external and internal irritations and characterized by red patches covered with white scales. When you scratch the patches, they begin to bleed. Infants and the elderly are rarely affected by psoriasis. However, when infants are afflicted, the disorder is usually very serious.

Psoriasis is not contagious, although many people think it is. It usually appears on areas of the head at the hairline, and on the ears, elbows, knees, back, and the region round the anus.

In treating psoriasis, it is helpful to include plenty of fish in your diet. It is also advisable to spend as much time as possible in the sun and fresh air.

The psychological aspect plays an important role in disorders of the skin. Therefore, it isn't surprising that psoriasis often starts when you are under a great deal of stress or have psychological conflicts. Think about your present situation. Is something trying to "get under your skin," has something that you wanted to keep at a distance gotten "too close for comfort," or are you "too thin-skinned"?

TREATMENT

● K 1—Yongquan
Kidney meridian, point 1
On the sole of the foot, from the middle furrow to the outside, level with the ball of the foot

● K 2—Rangu
Kidney meridian, point 2
On the inside of the foot, below the navicular bone

R 5–6 P.M.

Aromatic oil: bergamot

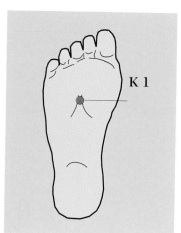

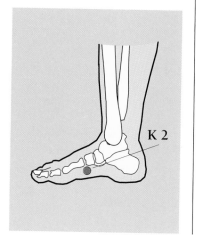

TREATMENT

● LI 15—*Jianyu*
Large-intestine meridian, point 15
On the extreme outside edge of the shoulder

● TW 3—*Zhongzu*
Triple-warmer meridian, point 3
On the basal joint of the ring finger

● B 60—*Kunlun*
Bladder meridian, point 60
On the heel

R 5–7 A.M., 3–5 P.M., 9–11 P.M.

Aromatic oils: chamomile, tea tree

Rheumatism

Rheumatism is a catchall word that describes many of the pains in the joints. Arthritis is a degenerative rheumatic illness (see page 34). In the early stages, the symptoms include restricted movement and tension. Later on, arthritis may cause joints to become painfully stiff.

Arthritis may be accompanied by a loss of appetite and of weight. It usually affects, in succession, the joints of the fingers, hands, shoulders, knees, feet, and hips. In the most serious cases, the patient ends up in a wheelchair.

Rheumatism of soft tissues does not affect the joints directly but attacks the tendons, nerves, and muscles surrounding them. The best-known example of this is tennis elbow (see page 75).

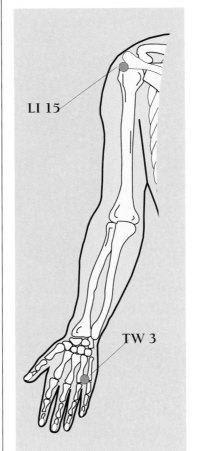

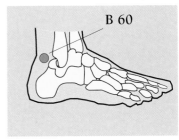

Sciatica

Sciatica is a term that usually describes the neuralgic pains that extend from the gluteal muscle into the leg and sometimes as far as the toes. In some cases, paralysis occurs. You can feel the pain of sciatica most clearly when you try to raise your leg while lying on your back. The primary causes are an irritation of the nerves or a slipped disk. Because of incorrect posture, the tissue of the disks is forced outward, pinching the sensitive nerves that run through the spinal column. The best prevention is regular exercise and correct posture when sitting and standing.

● G 30 —*Huantiao*
Gallbladder meridian, point 30
At the upper-inner end of the thighbone (femur)

● G 34—*Yanlingquan*
Gallbladder meridian, point 34
In the hollow next to the upper end of the fibula, on the outside

● G 43— *Xiaxi*
Gallbladder meridian, point 43
On the outside of the basal joint of the fourth toe

R 11 P.M.–1 A.M.

Aromatic oils: chamomile, sandalwood

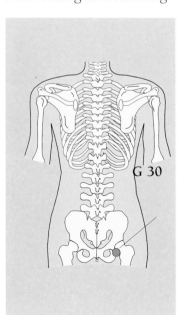

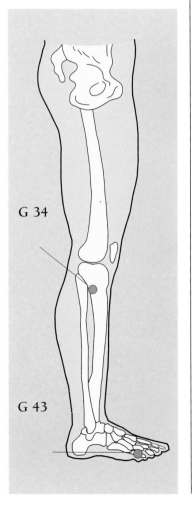

TREATMENT

● *LU 11—Shaoshang*
Lung meridian, point 11
On the inner joint of the thumb

● *LI 4—Hegu*
Large-intestine meridian, point 4
Press your thumb against your extended index finger, and you will see a bulge in the muscle. The highest point of the bulge is the acupressure point.

● *LI 2—Erjian*
Large-intestine meridian, point 2
On the second bone of the index finger

R 3–5 A.M., 5–7 A.M.

Aromatic oils: eucalyptus, chamomile

Sinusitis

Sinusitis is a painful inflammation of the cavities of the skull. Because the sinuses are connected to the nasal cavities, they are an easy target for the bacteria that enter the nose when we breathe.

The symptoms of sinusitis are fatigue, exhaustion, and headaches. Usually, the pain increases when you tilt your head down. In addition to acupressure, inhalations of chamomile and eucalyptus have proven to be effective remedies.

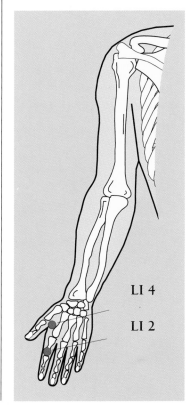

LI 4

LI 2

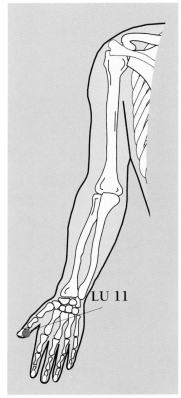

LU 11

Slipped Disk

Ever since humans started walking on two feet, the healthy spine has had a slight S curve to it.

Our posture mirrors our inner attitude. Some people are completely unstable inwardly and outwardly, and some people are "spineless."

The spine is very resilient. However, if there is too much strain, mentally or physically, or if such strain continues too long, we can develop back problems, ranging from a simple backache to sciatica, lumbago, or a slipped disk. Sometimes a slipped disk can keep a person in bed for weeks at a time and even cause temporary paralysis. In such cases, the body demands a period of rest and quiet. The pressure had become too great, and now the body (and mind) needs time to recuperate.

TREATMENT

● B 23—*Shenshu*
Bladder meridian, point 23
Between the second and third lumbar vertebrae

● B 25—*Dachangshu*
Bladder meridian, point 25
Between the fourth and fifth lumbar vertebrae

● B 31—*Shangliao*
Bladder meridian, point 31
In the hollow where the sacrum joins the pelvis

R 3–5 P.M.

Aromatic oil: rosemary

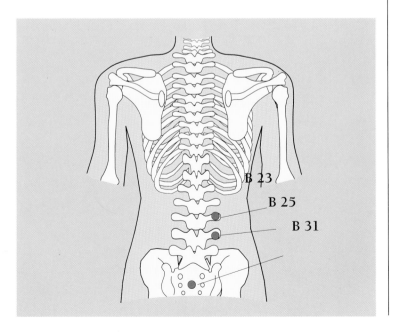

B 23

B 25

B 31

TREATMENT

● *LU 11—Shaoshang*
Lung meridian, point 11
On the inside of the first thumb joint

● *S 9—Renying*
Stomach meridian, point 9
On the side of the rise of the larynx

● *TW 1—Guanchong*
Triple-warmer meridian, points 1–3
On the nail joint of the ring finger

R 3–5 A.M., 7–9 A.M., 9–11 P.M.

Aromatic oil: sandalwood

Sore Throat

A sore throat can be a symptom of a cold or another illness. Tonsillitis and other infections can cause a sore throat. When a sore throat doesn't lead to a cold, you should consult your physician. From a psychological point of view, a sore throat indicates that you are no longer in a position to "swallow" things. This means you have to voice the annoyance and anger that you have been "swallowing." As long as you are only suffering from slight pain, you can achieve results quickly with acupressure.

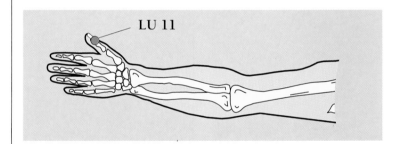

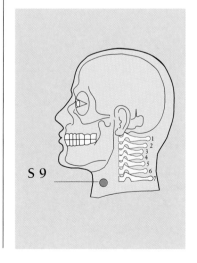

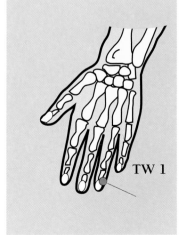

Stomach Disorders

The saying "I'm having trouble digesting that idea" shows how closely our stomach is related to our emotions. Stomach ulcers are often the result of years of anger and suppressed conflict. Stress produces excessive gastric acid, which, in turn, leads to a high level of acidity in the stomach and then to ulcers.

Although some things are "hard to digest," we keep our mouths shut and just "swallow" them. People with stomach problems often lack the self-confidence to solve their problems in a positive way. They have to learn to deal with their conflicts openly instead of turning their aggressions against themselves.

TREATMENT

● *S 24—Huaroumen*
Stomach meridian, point 24
To one side and above the navel

● *S 25—Tianshu*
Stomach meridian, point 25
*To one side between the navel
and the middle of the iliac bone*

● *S 36—Zusanli*
Stomach meridian, point 36
*On the outside of the shinbone
(tibia)*

R 7–9 A.M.

Aromatic oil: peppermint

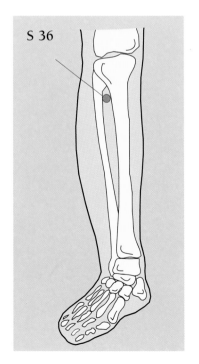

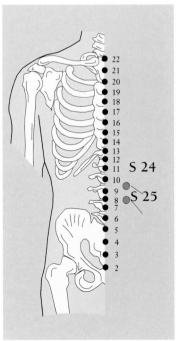

TREATMENT

Pain in the Upper Abdomen
● S 35—Dubi
Stomach meridian, point 35
The outside of the knee

● S 36—Zusanli
Stomach meridian, point 36
The outside of the shinbone
(tibia)

Diffuse Pain
● SP 4—Gongsun
Spleen-pancreas meridian,
point 4
The inside of the foot

● C 6—Neiguan
Circulation meridian, point 6
In the middle of the inside of
the forearm, the width of three
fingers below the bend of the
wrist

R 7–9 A.M., 9–11 A.M., 7–9 P.M.

Aromatic oil: fennel

Stomach Pains

We experience pain in the abdomen for many reasons. The pain can be due to indigestion, which results in flatulence, constipation, diarrhea, metabolic disorders, or cramps. However, it also can be caused by psychological stress. With young children and infants, abdominal pain is often a sign of the beginning of an infection or some other illness. Abdominal pains always should be taken seriously! Consult your doctor if you are not sure of the cause of the pain.

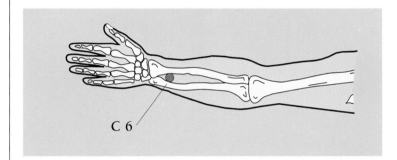

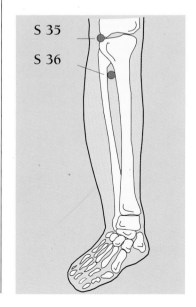

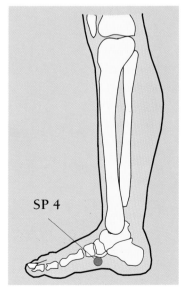

Tennis Elbow

You don't even have to step on a tennis court to suffer from tennis elbow. Tennis elbow is simply a clear sign of a strained elbow joint.

If repeated regularly and with some force, every movement of the arm can cause this kind of soft-tissue rheumatism. If you like do-it-yourself jobs or polishing your car weekends, you are just as likely to get tennis elbow as are people who put a lot of pressure on their arms in their jobs, such as secretaries, typists, and mechanics.

When you have tennis elbow, the tendons and muscles around your elbow joint also are affected. In the past, treatment required surgery, but, today, doctors restore the joint to health with an inconspicuous brace.

Acupressure eases pain and releases tension in the joints. In addition, it helps inflamed muscles and tendons heal sooner. However, even if you use acupressure, you have to ensure that the arm will not be strained again.

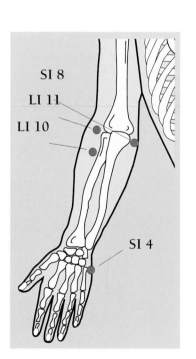

SI 8
LI 11
LI 10
SI 4

TREATMENT

● SI 4—*Wangu*
Small-intestine meridian, point 4
On the inner edge of the hand

● SI 8—*Xiaohai*
Small-intestine meridian, point 8
On the inside of the elbow joint

● LI 10—*Shousanli*
Large-intestine meridian, point 10
On the outside of the lower arm

● LI 11—*Quchi*
Large-intestine meridian, point 11
At the very end of the fold in the elbow

5–7 A.M., *R 1–3* P.M.

Aromatic oil: chamomile

TREATMENT

● *LI 4—Hegu*
Large-intestine meridian, point 4
Press your thumb against your extended index finger, and you will see a bulge in the muscle. The highest point of the bulge is the acupressure point.

● *TW 8 —Sanyanglo*
Triple-warmer meridian, point 8
The width of one hand above the bend of the wrist, between the ulna and radius

● *S 6—Jiache*
Stomach meridian, point 6
Above the masticatory muscle in front of the angle of the lower jaw (used mainly for pain in the upper jaw)

● *S 7—Xiaguan*
Stomach meridian, point 7
In the depression of the joint of the jaw(used mainly for pain in the lower jaw)

R 5–7 A.M., 7–9 A.M., 9–11 P.M.

Aromatic oil: clove

Toothache

Problems with the teeth usually symbolize suppressed aggressions and an unwillingness to make decisions. Grinding your teeth during the night is a certain sign that the subconscious is working intensely. Things that happened during the day but were repressed are now being digested. These are all those things that you had "to chew on" or problems that you had "to sink your teeth into."

Sometimes people have nightmares in which they suddenly lose all their teeth. The teeth are a symbol of vitality and strength; suddenly being without your teeth indicates a loss of vital energy. If you suffer frequently from toothaches, even though your dentist cannot find any cavities or signs of gum disease, you should examine your fears and anxieties.

Regardless of whether your toothache is psychological in nature or due to tooth decay, you can relieve the pain with acupressure.

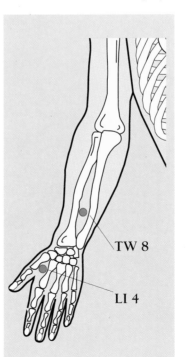

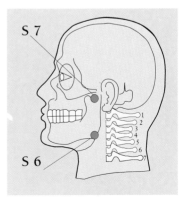

Treatments for Children's Disorders

Acupressure is suitable for children because it is very gentle. Increasing numbers of pediatricians are making use of natural healing methods. Some parents, too, are more open to natural ways of healing, using time-tested home remedies. Whether they use cold compresses around the legs to lower a fever, rub ointment on the child's chest, or prepare herbal inhalations, these parents understand the importance of not using a sledgehammer to open a pistachio nut. Instead, they are demonstrating their trust in the healing powers of nature.

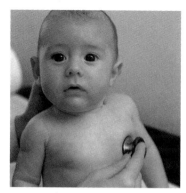

Many pediatricians trust natural healing methods.

Acupressure is a gentle and effective alternative treatment, especially for children who have adverse reactions to medications.

Pay Attention to Symptoms

With children, you have to be very careful, and you must take all symptoms seriously. Be sure not to wait too long before consulting a physician. On the other hand, don't worry too much, especially with young children and infants, if they are ill more often than you are. In the first few years, a child's immune system has to learn which foreign bodies are harmful and which are harmless. This learning process takes place only when the child has had all of the usual illnesses once. For example, after having measles or mumps, they are immune to them for the rest of their life.

The following is an overview of children's disorders that respond well to acupressure.

Anxiety

Anxiety can be a specific fear of certain people or events that seem to be threatening. It also can be based on something in a TV program the child has seen and cannot cope with, such as scenes of brutal violence or other aggressive action. Some thrillers, westerns, and science fiction films have been known to trigger extreme feelings of fear and anxiety. However, anxiety also can be triggered by dreams. This is especially difficult for children who are not old enough to articulate their feelings.

Acupressure provides a gentle and effective way to calm the child. You should spend a lot of time with your child and take any feelings of anxiety seriously. Talk to your child about anything that seems to be frightening or depressing him or her. Your loving care itself will have a relaxing effect.

TREATMENT

● H 3—*Shaohai*
Heart meridian, point 3
With the arm bent, at the inner end of the elbow bend

● H 7—*Shennen*
Heart meridian, point 7
In the bend of the wrist

● CV 19—*Houding*
Conception vessel, point 19
On the posterior fontanel of the head

R 11 A.M.–1 P.M.

Aromatic oil: tangerine

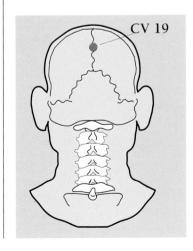

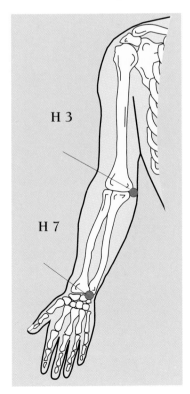

Apathy

Children who have trouble getting up in the morning, who generally need a lot of sleep, and who get tired very quickly suffer from a lack of energy. Acupressure can increase their level of activity and their overall joy in living, and it even can help them be more successful in school.

However, don't be too critical of a child who doesn't achieve the standards you set. Sometimes the standards are too high, and the child reacts to this pressure with a fear of failure and feelings of uncertainty. Such reactions also can occur when the child isn't getting enough parental love. The child's apathy forces the parents to pay attention to what is happening, even if this attention takes the form of criticism. Such feelings also can be a cause of bed-wetting (see page 80).

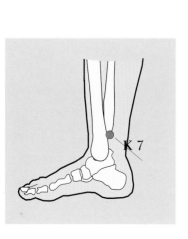

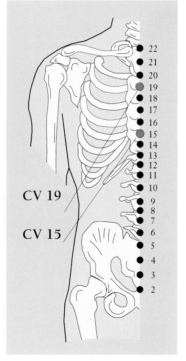

TREATMENT

● *CV 15—Jiuwei*
Conception vessel, point 15
On the lowest point of the breastbone

● *CV 19—Zigong*
Conception vessel, point 19
In the middle of the breastbone

● *K 7—Fuliu*
Kidney meridian, point 7
The width of three fingers above the outside of the ankle

S 7–9 P.M.

Aromatic oil: jasmine

TREATMENT

● *LU 9—Taiyuan*
Lung meridian, point 9
At the outer end of the bend of
the wrist

● *L 1—Dadun*
Liver meridian, point 1
In the corner of the big toenail

● *L 2—Xinjiang*
Liver meridian, point 2
At the basal joint of the big toe
when you spread your toes

R 1–3 A.M., 3–5 A.M.

Aromatic oil: sandalwood

Bed-Wetting

Bed-wetting is often a silent cry for help. You need to take it seriously. This is a way for the child to express psychological distress that he or she is unable to articulate.

Bed-wetting is also a way some children who lack sufficient love and affection are able to get the attention that they need. The fact that this attention is usually negative is beyond the control of the child. Of course, in a young child, all of this is taking place subconsciously.

Although bed-wetting is seldom caused by physical problems, you should consult your pediatrician, just to be sure.

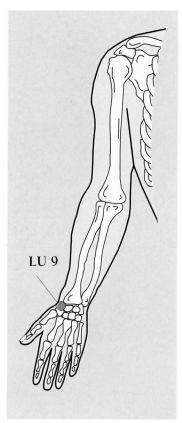

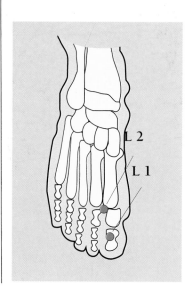

Fever

Fever is a condition in which the brain increases the body temperature. Usually, the increase in temperature is a reaction to the metabolic products of bacteria and inflammatory substances. An increase in temperature also can occur from sports activity, extreme exertion, and disorders of the part of the brain that regulates body temperature.

We generally consider a fever to be an oral temperature higher than 99.5°F (37.5°C) or a rectal temperature higher than 100.5°F (38°C). With infants, a rectal temperature higher than 101.3°F (38.5°C) is considered to be a fever.

Fever is one of the ways the body heals itself; however, if the fever does not go down by itself or with the help of cold compresses on the calves within a short time, you should consult your pediatrician, because fever can be a symptom of a more serious illness.

TREATMENT

● *GV 14—Dazhui*
Governing vessel, point 14
Between the seventh cervical vertebra and the first thoracic vertebra

● *LI 4—Hegu*
Large-intestine meridian, point 4
Press your thumb against your extended index finger, and you will see a bulge in the muscle. The highest point of the bulge is the acupressure point.

● *LI 11—Quchi*
Large-intestine meridian, point 11
On the outer end of the bend of the elbow

R 5–7 A.M.

Aromatic oils: bergamot, eucalyptus

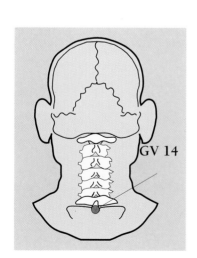

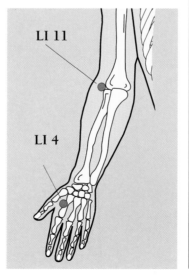

Flatulence

When children suffer from flatulence, they cry and complain. Acupressure can provide relief. Because there are various causes of flatulence—including stomach and intestinal disorders such as diarrhea and constipation, infections, indigestible food, and even swallowing air—you should consult your pediatrician if the symptoms persist.

TREATMENT

● *S 36—Zusanli*
Stomach meridian, point 36
On the outside of the shinbone (tibia)

● *SP 4—Gongsun*
Spleen-pancreas meridian, point 4
On the inside of the middle of the foot

● *CV 6—Qihai*
Conception vessel, point 6
Above the pubic bone

R 7–9 A.M., 9–11 A.M.

Aromatic oil: peppermint

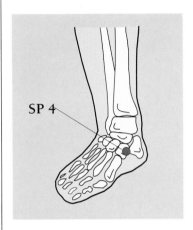

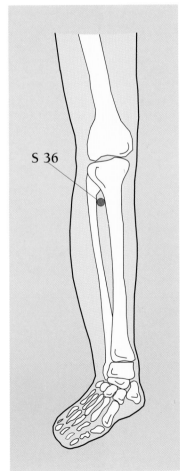

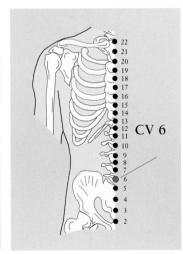

Restlessness and Nervous Conditions

Some children are overly nervous, suffering from sleep disturbances, hyperactivity, and excessive perspiration. They may be very pale or blush easily.

A restless or nervous child sometimes really whoops it up, overreacting to continual stimulation from the environment. Acupressure treatment can help, along with reducing the stimulation in the environment.

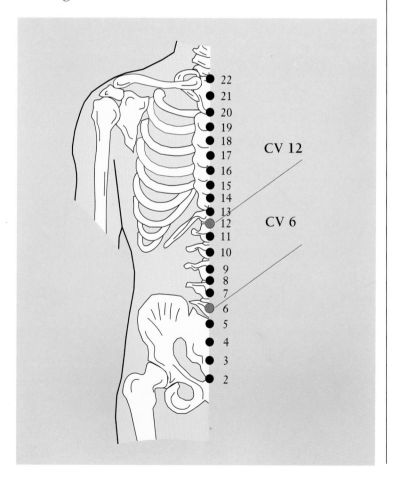

TREATMENT

● *CV 6—Qihai*
Conception vessel, point 6
Above the pubic bone

● *CV 12—Zhongwan*
Conception vessel, point 12
The width of four fingers above the navel

Sleeping Problems

All new parents dread another sleepless night because their baby is teething. Other parents aren't any happier when they have to cancel going to the movies because their child doesn't like the new babysitter. Sometimes children who have difficulty falling asleep lack harmony at home, or they have unfulfilled needs. They might suffer from anxiety. Using a soothing bedtime ritual every night can help in such cases.

However, if all the bedtime stories and lullabies do not help your child fall asleep, you should try acupressure. In no time, your child will drift off, and sleep deeply and restfully.

TREATMENT

● *S 36—Zusanli*
Stomach meridian, point 36
On the outside of the shinbone (tibia)

● *CV 4—Guanyuan*
Conception vessel, point 4
Above the pubic bone

R 7–9 A.M.

Aromatic oil: lavender

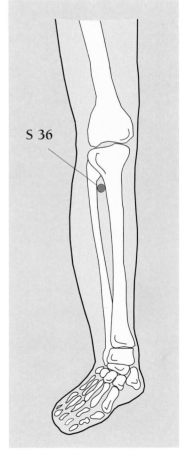

S 36

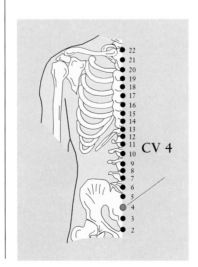

CV 4

Stuttering

Stuttering is not faulty pronunciation; it is an involuntary blocking or disruption of speech, and often can be hereditary.

Frequently stuttering is a psychological reaction to strain and conflict in the family. Stuttering may result when a child cannot cope with uncertainty and fears. The stuttering is then an expression of helplessness and of a lack of tranquility.

In many the cases, this speech disorder is slight. It also may be only a stage that will pass with time.

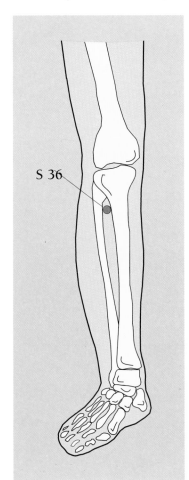

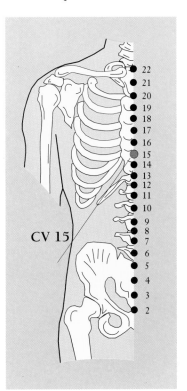

TREATMENT

● *S 36—Zusanli*
Stomach meridian, point 36
On the outside of the shinbone (tibia)

● *CV 15—Jiuwei*
Conception vessel, point 15
On the lowest point of the breastbone

R 7–9 A.M.

Aromatic oil: orange blossom

TREATMENT

Upper Jaw

● *LI 4—Hegu*
Large-intestine meridian, point 4
Press your thumb against your extended index finger, and you will see a bulge in the muscle. The highest point of the bulge is the acupressure point.

● *S 7—Xiaguan*
Stomach meridian, point 7
In the hollow of the joint of the upper jaw

R 5–7 A.M., 7–9 A.M.

Aromatic oil: clove

Lower Jaw

● *LI 4—Hegu*
See above.

● *S 6—Jiache*
Stomach meridian, point 7
Above the lower-jaw muscle

5–7 A.M., 7–9 A.M.

Aromatic oil: clove

Teething Problems

What parents can forget the long nights they were awake because their little one was howling from teething. Teething is a painful affair, and it influences the child's general well-being.

Most children get their first tooth, one of the middle incisors in the lower jaw, when they are about six months old. Next come the middle incisors in the upper jaw, and then the outer incisors in the upper and lower jaws. During the second year, the upper molars break through, followed by the canine teeth and the molars at the back of the jaw. However, the sequence does not have to follow any fixed timetable.

To make this painful process a little easier on children, treat them with these acupressure points. To bring on peaceful sleep, please refer to Sleeping Problems (page 84).

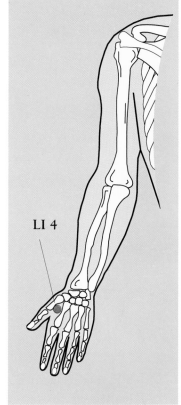

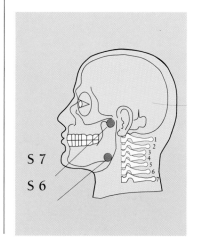

The Meridians—Points and Effects

The Bladder Meridian (Yang)

This meridian affects all the excretory organs. Use the points for problems involving the bladder and kidneys, hormonal difficulties, genital ailments, and pains occurring in the knees, feet, and back.

The most important acupressure points are the following:

● B1—Jingming (Eye Bright)
In the angle at the root of the nose
● B 23—Shenshu
Between the second and third lumbar vertebrae
● B 25—Dachangshu
Between the fourth and fifth lumbar vertebrae
● B 31—Shangliao (Upper Pit)
In the hollow formed by the sacrum on the skin of the back
● B 58—Feiyang (Upswing)
On the back of the calf
● B 60—Kunlun (Mountain in Tibet)
On the upper edge of the heel
● B 62—Shenmai
The width of two fingers below the ankle

The Circulation-Sexuality Meridian (Yin)

The acupressure points of this meridian affect sexuality and the circulation. Use the points in cases of circulatory problems, heart disorders, sleeplessness, and nervousness.

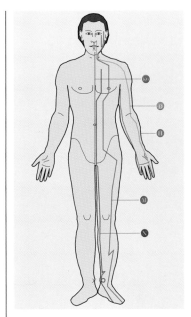

The most important meridians

The acupressure points of the bladder meridian apply to all urinary and genital ailments. They also work for hormonal difficulties and for disorders of the knees, feet, and back.

The most important acupressure point is the following:
● C 6—Neiguan (Inner Border)
In the middle of the lower part of the arm, between the ulna and radius, near the bend of the wrist

The Gallbladder Meridian (Yang)

The acupressure points of this meridian affect the psyche and are antispasmodic.

Use these points in cases of gallbladder complaints, pains in the shoulders and arms, lumbago, problems with knees and feet, headaches, disorders of the eyes, and nervousness. In most of these cases, apply pressure in a stimulating direction.

The most important acupressure points are the following:
● GB 20—Fengchi (Wind/Pond)
On the lower edge of the back of the head
● GB 24—Riyue (Sun/Moon)
Between the fifth and the sixth ribs
● GB 26—Daimai (Belt Vessel)
At the end of the twelfth rib
● GB 30—Huantiao (Jumping in the Hoop)
On the highest and innermost point of the thighbone (femur)
● GB 34—Yanglingquan (Yang Hill /Fountainhead)
In the hollow of the head of the fibula (on the side)
● GB 37—Guangming (Shining Brightness)
On the outside of the calf, the width of six fingers above the ankle
● GB 38—Yangfu (Yang Support)
On the outside of the calf, the width of five fingers above the ankle
● GB 40—Quixu (Hill/Market)
On the back of the foot

The points of the gallbladder meridian are nearly always applied in a stimulating way. They are most effective for the treatment of all kinds of pain in the joints.

● GB 43—Xiaxi (Tears/Descent)
On the back of the foot, to the side of the basal joint of the fourth toe

The Heart Meridian (Yin)

The heart meridian has a direct effect on the psyche and the autonomous nervous system. Stimulate the corresponding acupressure points in cases of nervousness, anxiety, depression, palpitations of the heart, excessive perspiration, circulatory disorders, and high blood pressure.

The most important acupressure points for these are the following:
● H 3—Shao Hai (Point of Joyful Living)
With the arm bent, on the inside of the bend in the elbow
● H 7—Shenmen (Spirit Gate)
In the outside of the bend of the wrist

The Kidney Meridian (Yin)

This meridian affects the metabolism. Stimulate it for urogenital disorders, impotence, menstrual problems, and ear complaints.

The most important acupressure point is the following:
● K 3—Taixi (Beginning of the Brook)
Between the highest point on the ankle and the Achilles tendon

"Point of Joyful Living" and "Spirit Gate" are the acupressure points on the heart meridian that control our psyche and the autonomous nervous system.

The Large-Intestine Meridian (Yang)

This meridian influences the functions of the mucous membranes. It also is related to excretion. Use these points for asthma, respiratory problems, lung complaints, and disorders of the intestines.

The most important acupressure points for these are the following:

● LI 4—Hegu (Meeting in the Valley)
Press your thumb against your extended index finger, and you will see a bulge in the muscle. The highest point of the bulge is the acupressure point.
● LI 10—Shousanli (Three Distances)
The width of three fingers below the bend of the elbow, on the outside
● LI 11—Quchi (Meandering Pond)
At the outer end of the bend of the elbow
● LI 15—Jianya (Shoulder Bone)
On the outer edge of the shoulder, in the hollow
● LI 20—Yingxiang (Welcoming Fragrance)
In the fold between the nose and the lips

As indicated by its name, the large-intestine meridian can ease disorders of the digestive system. You can use acupressure on these points also when you have respiratory problems.

The Liver Meridian (Yin)

The acupressure points of this meridian aid digestion. Use them for complaints of the liver and gallbladder and for depression, anxiety, and exhaustion.

The most important acupressure points are the following:
● LI 1—Dadun (Great Uprightness)
In the corner of the nail of the big toe
● LI 2—Xingjian (Gait/Route)
On the outer side of the splayed big toe

The Lung Meridian (Yin)

This meridian affects the respiratory tract and the skin. We apply pressure to its points for ailments of the throat and nose, such as pneumonia, bronchitis, asthma, colds, and runny nose, and for skin disorders. In addition, these points can help relieve pain in the wrist, elbow, and shoulder.

The most important acupressure points here are the following:
● LU 5—Chize (Pond of the Elbow)
In the middle of the bend of the elbow
● LU6—Kongzui
On the inner side of the forearm, the width of seven fingers above the bend of the wrist
● LU 7—Lieque (Bottleneck)
In the furrow between the ulna and radius
● LU 9—Taiyuan (Great Fountainhead)
At the end of the bend of the wrist, in the bend
● LU 11—Shaoshang (Dwindling Trade)
At the inner angle of the thumb

The lung meridian has to do with respiratory problems and skin disorders as well as all complaints that concern our relationship to the environment.

The Small-Intestine Meridian (Yang)

This meridian directly affects the mucous membranes and acts as an antispasmodic. You can use the acupressure points of the small-intestine meridian for problems with the shoulders and arms, diarrhea, intestinal problems, and nervousness.

The most important acupressure points are the following:
● SI 3—Houxi (The Rear Ravine)
Close your fist; at the end of the basal joint of the little fin-

ger, you will see a fold in the skin where you will find the acupressure point.

● SI 4—Wangu (The Fountainhead Point)

On the inside of the edge of the hand

● SI 7—Zhizheng (The Proper Link)

In the middle of the furrow between the wrist and the elbow

● SI 8—Xiaohai (The Small Sea)

On the outside of the elbow joint

● SI 11—Tianzong (Heavenly Ancestors)

In the center of the upper part of the shoulder blade

The Spleen-Pancreas Meridian (Yin)

The spleen-pancreas meridian is especially useful in cases of depression and anxiety.

This meridian affects the connective tissue of the entire body. You may use the corresponding acupressure points for all disorders of the stomach and intestines and for muscle ailments. In addition, these points influence the circulation of the blood and can help with menstrual problems, depression, and anxiety.

The most important acupressure points are the following:

● SP 1—Yinbai (The Hidden Place)

In the corner of the nail of the big toe

● SP 2—Dadu (Large City)

In the middle of the basal joint of the big toe

● SP 4—Gongsun (Grandson of the Prince)

In the middle of the inside of the foot

● SP 5—Shangqui (Consultation Hill)

Below the ankle

● SP 6—Sanyinjiao (Meeting Point)

The width of three fingers above the ankle

● SP 21—Dabao (Great Developer)

The Stomach Meridian (Yang)

This meridian influences the digestive system and the circulation. Additionally, it has a relaxing effect. Stimulate its points in cases of intestinal disorders or nervousness.

The most important acupressure points are the following:
● S 8—Touwei (Great Welcoming)
On the lower edge of the lower jaw
● S 9—Renying
On the elevation of the larynx
● S 24—Huaroumen (Smooth Flesh)
The width of two fingers below the navel
● S 25—Tianshu (Heavenly Pillar)
Between the navel and the pubic bone
● S 35—Dubi
When you bend your knees, on the outside of the resulting hollow
● S 36—Zusanli (Heavenly Serenity)
On the outside of the shinbone (tibia)
● S 41—Jiexi
In the middle of the tarsus

The triple-warmer meridian influences digestion, breathing, and urogenital functions.

The Triple-Warmer Meridian (Yang)

This meridian affects the digestive system, respiration, and the urogenital functions. Activate the acupressure points in cases of digestive problems, ear ailments, rheumatic pains, and pains in the shoulder, arm, and hand.

The important acupressure points are the following:
● TW 1—Guanchong (Point of Attack at the Border)
On the outer corner of the nail of the ring finger

● TW 3—Zhongzhu (Island in the Middle)
On the back of the hand
● TW 22—Erheliao (Corn on the Temples)
Above the zygomatic arch of the cheekbone, in front of the base of the ear

The Conception Vessel (Yin)

This vessel has its own energetic, functional circulation.

The most important acupressure points here are the following:
● CV 2—Qugu (Crooked Bone)
On the upper edge of the pubic bone
● CV 4—Guanyuan (Blocking the Border)
The width of two fingers above the pubic bone
● CV 6—Qihai (Sea of Energy)
The width of four fingers above the pubic bone
● CV 12—Zhongwan (Middle Channel)
The width of four fingers above the navel

The Governing Vessel (Yang)

This vessel has a psychological influence on the upper regions of the body and a physical effect on the lower regions of the body.

The most important acupressure points here are the following:
● GV 1—Changqiang (Growth of Strength)
At the end of the coccyx
● GV 12—Taodao (Path of Transformation)
Near the top of the spinal process
● GV 16—Naohu (Door to the Brain)
In the middle of the lower edge of the back of the head

In contrast to the meridians, the conception and governing vessels do not occur in pairs, and they run through the middle of the body.

About the Book

The Author

Dagmar-Pauline Heinke is a practitioner of acupressure, acupuncture, Ayurvedic medicine, and color therapy in Nürnberg, Germany. Heinke holds seminars on these subjects not only in Germany but also in Austria, Spain, France, Switzerland, and Turkey. She is especially concerned with the treatment of skin disorders and allergies.

Translation:Elfie Homann, Range Cloyd

Pictures

AKG, Berlin: 1,13; Archive Gerstenberg, Wietze: 21; IFA-Bilderteam, Muenchen: 4 (Comnet), 26 (Ostarhild); Ulrich Kerth, Muenchen: Cover (U1); Mainbild, Frankfurt: 23 (Schindler), U4; Alfred Pasieka, Hilden: 17; Claudia Rehm, Stockdorf: 28; Transglobe Agency, Hamburg: 76 (Jerrican/Charron); Tony Stone, Muenchen: 6 (Vera R. Storman), 12 (G. Brad Lewis), 19 (Zigy Kaluzny)

INDEX